Rec'd 11.28.05

For order information or questions, write or call:
   Re-visioning Professional Education: An Orientation to Teaching
   American College of Clinical Pharmacy
   3101 Broadway, Suite 650
   Kansas City, MO 64111
   816-531-2177
   816-531-4990 (Fax)
   accp@accp.com

Copyright © 2005 by the American College of Clinical Pharmacy. All rights reserved. This book is protected by copyright. No part of this publication may be reproduced, stored in a retrieval system, or transmitted, in any form or by any means, electronic or mechanical, including photocopy, without prior written permission of the American College of Clinical Pharmacy.

Printed in the United States of America.

Library of Congress Control Number: 2005932463
ISBN: 1-932658-27-0

Re-visioning Professional Education: An Orientation to Teaching

Thomas D. Zlatic, Ph.D.

Table of Contents

Preface: Re-visioning Professional Education: An Orientation to Teaching 1

Chapter 1: The Professional Nature of Teaching 5

Chapter 2: Re-visioning Professional Education 11

Chapter 3: Defining Critical Thinking within Professional Contexts 27

Chapter 4: Teaching Critical Thinking within Professional Contexts 47

Chapter 5: Holding a Cat by the Tail: Active Learning 61

Chapter 6: Using Assessment to Structure Learning: Putting It All Together 81

Chapter 7: Writing to Learn in Pharmacy Education 107

Works Cited 133

Index 147

Disclosure of Potential Conflicts of Interest 149

Acknowledgements

Thank you to the following reviewers for their critique of this publication.

Eric G. Boyce, Pharm.D.
Assistant Dean for Assessment and Professor of Pharmacy
School of Pharmacy
Wingate University
Wingate, North Carolina

Ina Lee Calligaro, Pharm.D.
Assistant Dean for Education
Associate Professor of Pharmacy Practice
Temple University School of Pharmacy
Philadelphia, Pennsylvania

Anne L. Hume, Pharm.D., FCCP, BCPS
Dean and Professor
College of Pharmacy
University of Rhode Island
Kingston, Rhode Island

Anne Y.F. Lin, Pharm.D.
Dean and Professor
College of Pharmacy-Glendale
Midwestern University
Glendale, Arizona

Therese Poirier, Pharm.D., M.P.H., BCPS, FCCP, FASHP
Professor and Associate Dean for Academic Affairs
Sourthern Illinois University Edwardsville
Edwardsville, Illinois

Mary T. Roth, Pharm.D., M.H.S., FCCP
Assistant Professor
Division of Pharmaceutical Policy and Evaluative Sciences
School of Pharmacy
University of North Carolina at Chapel Hill
Chapel Hill, North Carolina

Re-visioning Professional Education

Re-visioning Professional Education: An Orientation to Teaching

Preface

By now the scenario is familiar. The practice of pharmacy in the 21st century is responding to scientific/technological advancements and socioeconomic trends. Computers and robotics already have altered the distributive/dispensing functions performed by the pharmacist, and expert systems will continue to reduce or eliminate the pharmacist's need to perform pharmacokinetic calculations and to memorize drug properties and interactions. Pharmacy business systems based on microcomputers with bar coding and sophisticated data bases are streamlining operations, significantly reducing recordkeeping time. The growing number of pharmacy technicians, an increase in the use of mail-order pharmacy services, development of more self-care products, the ubiquity of the Internet, greater use of third-party payments, development and implementation of medication therapy management services, and the possibilities of physician dispensing and pharmacist prescribing will help to redefine the traditional role of a pharmacist. An increased need to relate to patients and to provide personal service will require pharmacists who are skilled in problem solving, decision making, and communication.

Pharmacy education has been pro-active in trying to shape future practice and in searching for ways to turn potential threats to traditional pharmacy practice into opportunities to enhance the profession and better serve society. It is clear that an evolving practice requires a parallel evolution in what is taught in pharmacy schools and how it is taught.

Changes in Society
⤵   ⤴
Changes in
Pharmacy Practice
⤵   ⤴
Changes in
Pharmacy Education

As in many disciplines, new pharmacy faculty often have had little or no formal training in teaching. There is a great deal for a new faculty member to know: constructing a syllabus, preparing lectures, writing exam questions, giving productive feedback, conducting discussion sessions, mentoring, creating an equitable grading system, balancing teaching with research and clinical activities, creating effective electronic materials and handouts, building confidence, working on committees, advising, and much more. Those will not be the topics of this book. Fortunately there are many good resources to help new practitioners become familiar with such basic topics and the strategies needed to enter the world of teaching.[1]

Although some practical tips will be provided within these pages, this is not so much a "how to" book as it is an orientation to pharmacy education—an attempt to get our bearings. Where are we? Where have we been? Where are we trying to go? Why are we trying to get there? What do we need to get there? The goal here is to be foundational or fundamental. Fundamental can mean "introductory" or "basic," as in a "clinical teaching for dummies" book. Rather, this book is meant to be foundational in the sense of providing a grounding for subsequent forays into techniques and strategies for becoming a successful teacher. It is an attempt to establish some coordinates, end points, and a few landmarks so we can avoid the proverbial trap of making great progress in the wrong forest. With such a goal, it is hoped that the audience will be not only new faculty but also other faculty interested in revitalizing their teaching. Coordinators of teaching initiatives might also use this book as a framework while they introduce junior faculty to educational techniques and strategies not covered here.

First, then, is an exploration of the nature of teaching. The book begins with the premise that teaching is based on fiduciary or covenantal relationships. In the absence of this orientation, pedagogical techniques and methods alone will not ensure arrival at the desired destination. Second, to prepare practitioners to provide pharmaceutical care, clinical educators must focus not only on teaching but also on learning. Presented here is a broad outline of contemporary pedagogical theory and practice, which includes reasons for incorporating higher order thinking into the pharmacy curriculum and a discussion of strategies for employing active learning so that students can attain educational goals related to the mission of pharmacy practice. The recommendation is to begin and end the educational process with ability outcomes: to identify what graduates must be able to do as a result of their education, to provide opportunities to practice those abilities, to establish criteria by which it can be determined how well students are performing the abilities, and to provide criteria-based assessment feedback so that students can improve. Undergirding this orientation is the fundamental assumption that professional education and general education must be integrated so that students are explicitly taught general abilities such as thinking, communication, and ethical decision making within professional contexts as they select/recommend drug therapy, educate patients, and collaborate with heath care providers. Because the attainment of these abilities requires appropriate attitudes, values, and habits, in addition to knowledge and skills, pharmacy educators need to ensure that all components of the abilities are practiced and assessed within the classroom and clinic. Integrating professional and general abilities can take pharmacy education beyond the traditional classroom and clinic so as to prepare 21st century practitioners who can respond to change and also envision the desired future, creating and implementing strategies to get there.

This book, rather than being innovative or groundbreaking, is more a distillation and application—and a remarkable display of chutzpah. Among other shortcomings of this volume is that the author is not a pharmacist, nor can I claim as a compensatory factor a degree in education. I apologize for the naïveté I may at times display, and I am appreciative of editors who have tried to weed out inanities. Nevertheless, there are some advantages. Sometimes the most valuable asset of a consultant is ignorance. Consultants in areas outside their own disciplines can be effective because they are ignorant of the rules, traditions, and methodologies of the people they are advising and therefore ask questions and propose solutions that would never occur to the more informed faculty ensconced in disciplinary thinking. New eyes can sometimes pick out things that the most trained eyes will overlook.

But more importantly, during 18 years within pharmacy education, I have been fortunate to work alongside extremely competent and motivated clinical faculty who have patiently taught me a great deal. At times I fear I am merely a ventriloquist's dummy for colleagues who in the early 1990s decided to take seriously the challenge to promote educational excellence in pharmacy, including Michael Maddux, Dimitra Vrahnos Travlos, Sheldon Holstad, Jack Burke, and Robert E. Smith. Students and residents subjected to these early innovations later as faculty helped to refine and extend an ability-based approach to teach and assess students, and I continue to learn much from them: Mary Roth McClurg, Wafa Dahdal, Trish Berry, Brenda Thompson Gleason, Sara Schroeder Lanfear, Brian Seiz, Jennifer Kasair Whaley, Keri Mattes Sims, and others. Outside of pharmacy we were fortunate to have resource persons available to suggest possibilities and provide assistance, including Charles Bonwell, Eric Hobson, Peter Hurd, and Gary Rolison. Working with American Association of Colleges of Pharmacy members on committees and projects has been very educational and rewarding. Particularly influential were five years of implementation of a Foundation for the Improvement of Post-Secondary Education (FIPSE) grant in collaboration with Holly Mason, Dana Purkerson Hammer, Gary Hollenbeck, Susan Meyer, the remarkable Bob Chalmers, and Georgine Loacker and other faculty from Alverno College. I have learned a great deal from collaborative projects with scholars such as John Nichols, Eric Boyce, Diane Beck, Deanne Nowak, Trudy Banta, Catherine Palumbo, faculty from Alverno College, and others. As participant and presenter of numerous pedagogical workshops, I have been impressed with the dedication that pharmacy faculty display toward a quest for educational excellence. And I am appreciative of current colleagues willing to undertake innovative approaches to meeting new challenges. Special thanks to those who assisted in the revision of this manuscript, including Michael Maddux, Mary Roth, Brenda Gleason, Peter Hurd, Jack Burke, and Susan Mueller. And of course without Mary Lou Zlatic there would be little reason to undertake anything.

Some of the chapters here have been previously published in different forms. Appreciation is extended to those who gave permission to rework and republish these materials. Chapter Two in part is adapted from an article from the *Journal of Pharmacy Practice*. Versions of Chapters Three, Four and Five were published in *Critical Thinking in Pharmacy Education: A Sourcebook*, which was enabled in part by a Gateway Award for Pharmacy Schools (GAPS) Grant administered by the American Association of Colleges of Pharmacy (AACP). Chapters Six and Seven are based upon two articles that appeared in the *Journal of Pharmacy Teaching*. My appreciation as well to the reviewers who provided both criticism and encouragement for an earlier manuscript of this work; of course they are not to be held responsible for any problems that still appear.

Notes

1. For instance, Lucas CJ, Murry JW Jr. New faculty: a practical guide for academic beginners. New York: Palgrave Publishers Ltd, 2002. Filene PG. The joy of teaching: a practical guide for new college instructors. Chapel Hill: University of North Carolina Press, 2005. Boice R. Advice for new faculty members: nihil nimus. Boston: Allyn and Bacon, 2000. Lowman J. Mastering the techniques of teaching. San Francisco: Jossey-Bass, 1984.

Chapter 1: The Professional Nature of Teaching

Teaching is a profession.

To be successful in that profession one needs to be concerned about outcomes, methods, strategies, and techniques. But it is important first to understand the obligations that stem from the professional nature of teaching. Pharmacy educators have an advantage here because of their professional education and experience.

The Profession of Pharmacy

All in the medical fields can recognize distinguishing traits of a professional, among others: advanced education, a sophisticated body of knowledge, membership in an organization that has formulated and adopted a code of a conduct and that has self-policing responsibilities, a service orientation, and a covenantal bond with patients. This last one, a covenantal bond, gets close to the essence of professionalism: the essential trait of a professional has to do with relationships.

In 1996, William Zellmer asked whether pharmacy was an occupation or a profession.[1] At that time he concluded pharmacy was an occupation on its way to becoming a profession. His reasoning was that pharmacy traditionally was a product-oriented discipline. When the primary mission of pharmacy practice was to prepare and dispense medications, the primary attention of the pharmacist was to a product. With the advent of pharmaceutical care as an explicit mission of pharmacy practice, pharmacy began to evolve toward a patient-oriented discipline. One can argue persuasively that pharmacy has been a profession for a long time, but it is that transition from a product-centered ethos toward a patient-centered ethos that intensifies the professional nature of pharmacy.[2]

Of course, definitions are stipulative and variable. "Profession" covers a wide variety of careers and practices. Professional actors, professional sports players, professional carpet cleaners. Those are appropriate but different uses of the term "professional" than is being employed when we say, "pharmacy is a profession" or "teaching is a profession." Again, that difference hinges on relationships—the types of relationships that the professional establishes with the persons that he or she serves.

That difference is encoded in the language we commonly use to refer to those relationships. Faculty drill into students that they should refer to people who come into chain pharmacies as "patients," not "customers." But students do not always understand the implications of the terminology. In an occupation, the people that we work with are customers. Toward them, of course, we have legal and ethical responsibilities, but our primary obligation is not to the customer but to the person who employs us. Working in the best interests of the customer is often an effective strategy for promoting the best interests of the company, but our primary responsibility is to the company, to our stockholders and employers. With the customer we have a financial or mercantile relationship. When I buy tires, I know that the salesperson is likely to recommend a product that not only meets my needs but also produces the biggest profit. If I ask a salesclerk at a department store how the expensive pink plaid suit I am trying on looks, I know I must be cautious when she says, "It's perfect, sir; it makes you look ten years younger." *Caveat emptor.*

In a profession we do not have customers. In medicine we have patients. In law we have clients. In religion we have a flock or congregation or parishioners. And in teaching we have students. This is not, or should not be, a simple matter of semantics.

If a doctor pokes her head out of an examining room to ask the nurse, "How many more customers do we have in the waiting room?" most likely the doctor will have one fewer if a patient happens to overhear the comment. If a preacher from the pulpit surveys his congregation smilingly and mutters under his breath into an open microphone that he does not know is on, "excellent—a lot more customers tonight," the faithful may feel a little awkward in responding to common prayer.

Professionals do not have customers. Instead the relationship they have with the people they serve is one of trust. They have fiduciary obligations toward the persons whom they serve. A fiducial relationship is a "faith" relationship, a convenantal relationship (fiduciary, from L. *fides*, meaning faith). In this sense, a professional is someone who has special knowledge that is important for our well being. It is a complex knowledge that usually we cannot understand, and we cannot easily evaluate the services of the provider. We cannot know if it is truly needed and sometimes we cannot evaluate even whether it has been successful. Instead, we must trust the professional. As a practical matter it is wise to do research and to get second opinions, of course, but ultimately we say in effect, I must give you, the professional expert, the gift of trust. And the professional, in turn, promises to act in our best interest: the professional's first responsibility is to us.

This is the ideal, and one not always exemplified in practice. There are professionals who behave unprofessionally. But it is in the violations of fiduciary responsibility that we see how essential it is. Unfortunately we have been accustomed to all sorts of heartless scams in society at large, but we are still appalled when we hear of a dentist who puts metal caps on the teeth of every student in a first-grade class of Hispanic children because the government allows him $35 for every tooth he treats, knowing that their parents are not likely to protest since many are illegally in the country and afraid to cause trouble. Our horror and repulsion when we hear of televangelists raking in contributions or of clergy abusing children come not only from the heinous actions themselves but also from the dashed expectations we had for the highly trusted professionals who perform them. If patients must worry that the only reason a doctor tells them they must have liver surgery is that his 18-year-old daughter is about to enroll in an expensive university, rational medical care will crumble. Society cannot function without the expectation of trust, of fiduciary obligations, from professionals.

The Profession of Teaching

Teaching is a profession. It is based upon fiducial relationships between teachers and students.

Thus it is trivializing and demeaning to suggest that "students are our customers"—demeaning both to students and to faculty. This is not to impugn the motives of those who speak those words. Usually the intentions are noble. What they are urging is that students be treated with respect, that they be placed at the center of educational decision making—which they should. Sometimes in higher education, unfortunately, under pressures of teaching and research demands, the temptation may be to view students as unfortunate interruptions in our academic lives; in some cases teaching may be viewed as the price we must pay in order to conduct research. Or worse, students sometimes are treated brusquely or insensitively when they seek assistance.

The slogan "students are our customers" is an effort to curtail such abuses. The problem is not that the customer model places expectations too high on the way we should treat students; the problem is that it sets the expectations too low. Our obligations to our students run much deeper than our obligations to any customers, no matter how highly valued they are. As in pharmacy practice, we have with students not primarily an economic but rather a fiducial relationship.

Furthermore, the metaphor is not merely misleading; it is dangerous. In the business world, the truism that "the customer is always right" is cynical. It does not mean working in the best interests of customers; it means keeping them happy. Grade inflation, watered-down courses, and completely elective curricula can be protective strategies to ensure that student customers walk away from courses feeling they got their money's worth.

Paternalism in any profession must be avoided. Students should be allowed to make choices, and student evaluation and feedback are important factors in program enhancement. But without a holistic understanding of a discipline, students often are not in a position to make trustworthy judgments about what is necessary to learn to enter a profession. Designing courses to attract students in the way marketers position a product is the "academic equivalent of ambulance chasing."[3]

More disturbing is the distortion that a consumer paradigm for education creates for how we envision and conduct the educational enterprise. Paradigms are very powerful because they are often "invisible"; when unacknowledged and unexamined, paradigms can shape our attitudes, opinions, and behavior in subtle ways without our being aware of it. The customer model, even when well-intentioned, insinuates that education is a commodity to be purchased. Learning is reduced to knowledge consumption, a rapid acquisition of facts. This attitude is reflected in a common student complaint about being required to participate in collaborative or problem-based learning: "I'm paying you to teach me."

Education as reflection, as expansion of a world view, or as development of complex abilities is more difficult to justify in this environment. The wise instructor in such an educational model will avoid controversial or challenging positions that might upset the customers. Taking neutral positions and skirting topics that might challenge students' opinions or comfort level are tactics consistent with sound marketing principles. The notion of a professor as someone who "professes," who speaks out and takes a stand, is replaced by the concept of a professor as shrewd analyzer of exit polls. If the customer model prevails, "teaching for tips" might be one outcome of a customer model of education.[4]

The problem then with a consumer model of education is not that it puts too much emphasis on the student, but that it does not go far enough. The alternative view, that we have fiducial responsibilities to the people we "serve," means our primary obligation as teachers is to our students, collectively and as individuals. Their success determines our success. Of course teachers have multiple obligations—to the college, the profession, one's discipline, society—and an ethical balance must be achieved among all of them, but the first and primary obligation is to students: to do our best to motivate and encourage them to learn; to assist them to develop the knowledge, skills, and attitudes they need to perform successfully in their homes, professions, and communities; and to try to instill in them a desire and ability to become lifelong, self-directed learners. This orientation is more important than the methodologies and strategies we choose to employ.

Orienting Ourselves to Teaching

There is no one mold or formula for a successful teacher, nor should there be.[5] Faculty have different personalities, strengths, disciplines, and goals; students have multiple interests, learning styles, and needs. But although style, technique, and persona may vary, some broad commonalities often distinguish an excellent teacher.

In a variety of workshops over the years I have asked participants to think about the best teachers they ever had and to define the characteristics that made them so. To devise a mnemonic, in the workshops we always tried to convert answers into "c" words, for instance, "clear," "comedic," "clever," "conscientious," "courteous," etc. But three important traits recur again and again—all of which dovetail into professionalism.

Caring. This is the most common response, first in frequency and in importance. The excellent instructor creates a learning environment that is nurturing and safe. "It was clear that the instructor cared whether I learned or not." "The instructor went out of his/her way to make sure I got it." "I tried hard because I did not want to let the teacher down." "I never felt embarrassed about asking a question." "I never would have made it, but she kept insisting I could do it, and showed me how."

Competent. The excellent teacher is an expert, someone who knows both the material and how to present it. "The guy is an encyclopedia." "We used to sit around trying to come up with questions to stump her." "Her handouts and lectures were always clear and organized." "He could explain things to me in ways I could understand."

Challenging. Caring and competent sometimes are enough to justify the label of "a good teacher." But a "best" or excellent teacher often entails the third most common characteristic: challenging. "She taught me how to study." "He motivated me to maximize my potential." "He made me want to learn." "She taught me how to think." Frequently, appreciation for a challenging teacher is delayed. It is remarkable how many people say that at one time the best teacher they ever had was also initially the worst. The teacher was unreasonable, unhelpful, they thought, never satisfied, always pushing. "I hated her" is a common response, often expressed with a sheepish grin. Once these students recognized that the reason the instructor challenged them was that he or she cared enough about them to risk their displeasure, they responded with what often turned out to be lifelong appreciation.

All of this of course is anecdotal, and individual students often respond differently. But it is striking how frequently the excellent teacher is described as a gifted person with high standards who motivates students to achieve by taking a personal interest in them, and by providing not only intellectual guidance but also emotional support and encouragement. All three traits are essential. Being challenging without being caring produces alienation. Being caring without being competent produces frustration.

What this suggests is that like any ability, the ability of teaching is an integration of knowledge, skills, and attitudes. Being a good teacher means a cultivation of each.

Parker Palmer in *The Courage to Teach* says that too often discussions about improving teaching focus on what we should teach, how we should teach, or why we should teach, but seldom on the most important question, who the person is that teaches.[6] His thesis is that *"good teaching cannot be reduced to technique; good teaching comes from the identity and integrity of the teacher"*(10). In teaching, delivery of fact and training in methodologies and skills are important. Knowing how to motivate and inspire students is at least as important. Demonstrating integrity and faithfulness is foundational.

In philosophy a distinction is made between two types of ethics: ethics of action and ethics of character. The first is concerned with deciding what is the right thing to *do* in a particular situation; ethical theories such as deontology and utilitarianism provide guidelines for correct behavior. Ethics of character on the other hand asks, What type of person must I *be*, and what characteristics or virtues must I possess? The difference has important implications for pharmacy professionals providing pharmaceutical care, as they care for and care about people with whom they have formed fiduciary relationships.

The same can be said for teaching professionals. "What must I do to be a good teacher?" is an important question. "What type of person must I be to be a good teacher?" is a more foundational one. We need always to begin with the correct orientation before we attempt to follow any map, no matter how accurate and detailed.

Questions for Reflection

1. Who was the best teacher you have had, and why?
2. What are your goals in teaching?
3. In your experience, did most teachers demonstrate fiduciary obligations?
4. How would you answer, "What must I do to be a good teacher?"
5. How would you answer, "What type of person must I be to be a good teacher?"

Notes

1. Zellmer WA. Searching for the soul of pharmacy. Am J Health Syst Pharm 1996;53:1911-6.
2. See Reich WT. What care can mean for pharmaceutical ethics. J Pharm Teach 1996;5:1-17.
3. These issues are discussed by Ong WJ. Presidential address 1978: the human nature of professionalism. PMLA 1979;94:385-94.
4. See Sajé N. Teaching for tips. Liberal Educ 2005;91:48-51.
5. For a discussion of a variety of teaching modes or styles, see Reinsmith WA. Archetypal forms in teaching: a continuum. Westport, CT: Greenwood Press, 1992.
6. Palmer PJ. The courage to teach: exploring the inner landscape of a teacher's life. San Francisco: Jossey-Bass Publishers, 1998:4.

Chapter 2: Re-visioning Professional Education

> It is remarkable how easily and insensibly we fall into a particular route, and make a beaten track for ourselves. I had not lived there [at Walden Pond] a week before my feet wore a path from my door to the pond-side; and though it is five or six years since I trod it, it is still quite distinct. It is true, I fear that others may have fallen into it, and so helped to keep it open. The surface of the earth is soft and impressible by the feet of men; and so with the paths which the mind travels. How worn and dusty, then, must be the highways of the world, how deep the ruts of tradition and conformity!
>
> *Henry David Thoreau, Walden*

When Henry David Thoreau in the 1840s decided that the pace of life in America had become too fast, he retreated to Walden Pond, where for two years he observed and reflected in order to discover and reorient himself to what was most essential in life. One genius of Thoreau was his ability to extract deep meaning from everyday observation: Be careful with your facts, he advised, you never know when one will "flower into a truth." The truth in the epigraph above is that often we can become imprisoned by our mental models. The ease and speed of the more-traveled path closed Thoreau's eyes or will to different routes or even different destinations. Models, or paradigms, are essential for understanding reality, but when used unreflectively, the models darken as well as enlighten. They open up some possibilities for understanding while closing down other options.

As a trivial example, try this simple task:

> Remove six letters for a paradigm shift:
> a s p i a r a x d i l e g t m t s h e i f r t s

The simple task is difficult only if we are unable to shake the concept that "six letters" refers to six discrete letters rather than to the phrase "six letters."

> a spi araxdi l e g t m t sheif r t s
> a S p I a r a X d i L E g T m T s h E i f R t S
> a   p ara di   g   m sh   if t

Along the same lines, identify the mistakes:

> There are three errers in
> in this sentence.

Those who can solve the riddle and identify the errors must be able to move from chirographic mistakes (misspelling of "errors" and repetition of "in") to the semantic level. The third error is at the level of meaning: the third error is that there are only two errors in the sentence!

In education, mental models and paradigms are also extremely influential, laying the groundwork for what we want to accomplish, how we want to accomplish it, and the means by which we evaluate whether or not we have accomplished it. Such models enable us to identify and organize data and assign value or importance, but they can also blind us to alternative approaches that are irreconcilable with the paradigm.

One motivation for the Pharm.D. as the sole entry-level degree was an evolution in the mission of pharmacy practice. Pharmacists for years scrupulously had fulfilled their primary mission of preparing and dispensing medications. With changes in society, science, technology, and the health care environment, the mission of pharmacy became more complex: providing pharmaceutical care and taking responsibilities for drug therapy outcomes. In 2004 the Joint Commission of Pharmacy Practitioners reached a consensus on a vision of the profession in 2015: "Pharmacists will be the health care professionals responsible for providing patient care that ensures optimal medication therapy outcomes."[1] This implies an increasing need for interprofessional collaboration with other practitioners in the health professions.

There is a larger context. In 1999 the Institute of Medicine (IOM) identified a crisis resulting from a "broken health care system" in the United States that was spawning widespread overuse, misuse, and underuse of services.[2] As a corrective, in "Health Professions Education: A Bridge to Quality," the IOM proposed its own vision toward which health professions should strive: "*All health professionals should be educated to deliver patient-centered care as members of an interdisciplinary team, emphasizing evidence-based practice, quality improvement approaches, and informatics.*" The IOM's evaluation that "Education for the health professions is in need of a major overhaul," prompted its recommendation for an educational restructuring focused on six overarching competencies common to all health professionals: provide patient-centered care, work in interdisciplinary teams, employ evidence-based practice, apply quality improvement, utilize informatics.[3]

The expanded vision and mission for pharmacy practice entail a different mission for pharmacy education as well. That mission is to prepare graduates to provide pharmaceutical care: to care for and to care about patients while taking responsibility for their drug therapy outcomes. To accomplish that mission, pharmacy education must adapt both to the emerging competencies required in the health professions and to contemporary educational theories and practices. The recommended transformation in health education by IOM and others will require cooperation at many levels within the professions and institutions of higher learning. Here we will focus more on what individual instructors can do to contribute to the preparation of practitioners functioning in new roles within new models of health care delivery. In later chapters we will address current educational topics such as active learning, higher order thinking, assessment as learning, and ability-based education, but first we should consider alternative paradigms for education.

Teaching Paradigm and Learning Paradigm

In a highly influential article, Robert Barr and John Tagg proposed two paradigms of education: a teaching paradigm and a learning paradigm. The authors suggested that students in the 21st century can be better prepared if educators adopt the Learning Paradigm, in which "a college's purpose is not to transfer knowledge but to create environments and experiences that bring students to discover and construct knowledge for themselves, to make students members of communities of learners that make discoveries and solve problems."[4]

As a heuristic strategy, we can associate the teaching paradigm with the earlier mission of pharmacy education: training students to prepare and dispense medications. And we can associate the learning paradigm with the current mission of pharmacy education: to prepare students to provide pharmaceutical care.

First we must acknowledge the inevitable oversimplification from any such binary divisions. In reality, the pedagogical situation is much more complex; in most cases a continuum rather than a bifurcation would be a more accurate representation. But nonetheless, for illustrative purposes, we can chart out educational approaches and strategies as they relate to the missions of pharmacy practice.

Old Mission: Preparing/Dispensing	**Current Mission: Pharmaceutical care**
Teaching Paradigm	*Learning Paradigm*
Stored Knowledge Model	Constructed Knowledge Model
Content-centered	Ability-centered
Instructor-oriented	Student-oriented
Didactic Teaching	Active/Experiential Learning
Professional Training	Professional Education

In a stored knowledge model of learning, brains are containers to be filled with data. The instructor's job is to do the filling. Facts flow from the mind of the instructor through the vocal cords across the airwaves and become deposited, unaltered, through the ears and into the minds of the students. There the facts are layered on top of one another, filed for later retrieval. Because of limited space, we may have to refuse to learn some things because only so many facts can fit.

In a teaching paradigm, particularly when conjoined with a stored knowledge model of learning, the focus is on the instructor. Delivery of content is the primary goal of the instructor. Faculty development programs focus on helping instructors to prepare informed, clear, organized, interesting lectures with masterful handouts and illuminating Power Point™ slides. And if transmission of knowledge is the primary goal and if teaching is the focus of the educator's activity, then such preparation is an appropriate strategy.

Teaching the material does not always coincide with student learning. Probably many experienced teachers have pretended not to see a student hand raised in question because the teachers knew that any interruption would preclude finishing the presentation of all the material. Such compulsion is understandable. Committed to our discipline and to excellence in education, we feel guilty if we do not get across all the important content.

This is where a paradigm shift can be helpful. Should our commitment be more to teaching than to learning, to the

> ... a college's purpose is not to transfer knowledge but to create environments and experiences that bring students to discover and construct knowledge for themselves, to make students members of communities of learners that make discoveries and solve problems.
>
> *Barr and Tagg*

content more than to the student? Is it more important to present all the material, or for the students to understand it?

A constructed knowledge model proposes instead that learners do not simply receive knowledge but construct it. Our minds are not *tabulae rase* or empty boxes. We all have our individual preconceptions and misconceptions that can both advance and impede learning. In addition, learning is not only a cognitive but also a psychological and emotional activity; motivations and goals, for instance, play a crucial role. Further, it is apparent that different students have different learning styles: what works for one will not necessarily work for another. Some may be more audile or visual in learning; some may require hands-on learning; some may shy away from confrontational learning strategies such as debates. The constructed knowledge model places more emphasis on these differences in individual students and more emphasis on flexibility in approaches to assist them in their learning.[5]

In a learning paradigm the focus switches from the instructor to the student, from content to abilities, from passive learning to active learning. What the instructor does is of course extremely important, but it is what the student does that becomes the indicator of educational success. The instructor plans classes and courses with an understanding of a need to adapt to a number of learning styles and is willing to modify course activities in response to student and other assessment feedback.

Content remains extremely important, but it is put into the service of abilities. The goal of education in this model is not simply to produce knowledge, but to enable students to integrate knowledge, skills, attitudes, and values so that they can perform clearly defined abilities, such as thinking, communication, ethical decision-making, selecting and monitoring drug therapy, and educating health care professionals. Abilities cannot be developed without practice, and thus active learning is an important strategy in a learning paradigm. Lectures are still valuable, but they are only one tool for developing student abilities.

Again, one can emphasize too much the exclusivity of these contrasts. The sketches above are more caricatures than realistic snapshots. Nonetheless, it can be helpful to see the changes in pharmacy preparation in terms of an increasing attention to education over training. Training and education overlap but are different. Training involves teaching people the correct ways of thinking, acting, and valuing. Training is an important component of professionalization. Pharmacy students are trained to put labels on medicine bottles correctly, to respond appropriately in common patient interactions, to calculate creatinine clearance, to demonstrate empathy, to value collaboration. And through a carefully planned process of socialization, pharmacy students can be trained to act and look like pharmacists.

It is becoming increasingly clear that such training and application are insufficient for contemporary practice. With the mission of pharmaceutical care, pharmacy graduates "need to be more than just professional problem solvers who come in, recite the solution, and leave like technological mercenaries. They must not only solve problems, but frame them."[6]

Graduates must be enabled to solve not only problems whose solutions are known but also problems whose solutions are not known. They not only must learn the "right" way of thinking, acting, and valuing within their profession, but they also must develop the facility to question and evaluate what they learn and to develop new ways of thinking, acting, and valuing. This is what education provides over and above training. Education involves critical abilities to evaluate and challenge "correct" ways of doing things, to respond to novel situations, to modify procedures, to make judgments, to innovate. Critical thinkers learn to notice and reflect upon paradigms—to find not only a different path to the pond but maybe totally new ponds.

One goal of this book is to promote the integration and development of general and professional abilities within a student-centered, active learning environment. Professional education should involve the exercise of general abilities within professional contexts. Taking pharmacy education beyond the clinic and beyond the traditional classroom is necessary to see that professional education is the exercise of general abilities such as thinking and communicating within professional contexts.

Integrating Professional and General Education

In light of external pressures such as accreditation, and in response to internal motivations to improve education, many colleges of pharmacy have structured their curricula around ability outcomes that students should demonstrate in order to graduate. To facilitate this process, in 1994 the American Association of Colleges of Pharmacy (AACP) Center for Advancement of Pharmaceutical Education (CAPE) published *Educational Outcomes*, with general and professional ability outcomes segregated in this way:[7]

General Ability Outcomes	**Professional Ability Outcomes**
Thinking	Provide pharmaceutical care
Communication	Manage the practice
Valuing and ethical decision making	Manage medication use systems
Social and contextual awareness	Promote public health
Social responsibility	Provide drug information and education
Social interaction	
Self-learning abilities	

Including general outcomes within a set of expectations for pharmacy graduates was a forward-thinking move, but a problem with creating two discrete sets of goals is that it can imply that the general and professional outcomes should be addressed at different parts of the curriculum or that separate learning activities must be created in order to develop each set of abilities. The separate delineations of general and professional ability outcomes can obscure the intimate connections between them. This is one reason that the 2004 CAPE outcomes attempted to integrate general and professional outcomes. For instance, Pharmaceutical Care, one of three terminal ability outcomes for pharmacy graduates, is described this way:

> Provide pharmaceutical care in cooperation with patients, prescribers, and other members of an interprofessional health care team based upon sound therapeutic principles and evidence-based data, taking into account relevant legal, ethical, social, economic, and professional issues, emerging technologies, and evolving pharmaceutical, biomedical, sociobehavioral, and clinical sciences that may impact therapeutic outcomes.[8]

> [Pharmacy graduates] need to be more than just professional problem solvers who come in, recite the solution, and leave like technological mercenaries. They must not only solve problems, but frame them.
>
> *AACP 1988 Academic Affairs Committee*

The outcome statement incorporates knowledge and perspectives from several disciplines, and subdivisions of the statement attempt to connect the professional ability to general outcomes. For instance, under "Provide Patient Care" it is clear that higher order or critical thinking is necessary to provide pharmaceutical care:

"Retrieve, analyze, and interpret the professional, lay, and scientific literature to provide drug information to patients, their families, and other involved health care providers." Nonetheless, some are concerned that the responsibility to teach general abilities in pharmacy courses may appear less obvious because they are not explicitly singled out as outcomes.[9]

The nature of the interconnections between general and professional education has been debated since at least 1868 when it was proposed that [t]he very first thing after good moral principle in a young man is a liberal education. ...When we start to improve our profession, let us begin by insisting on a better preliminary education, the basis not only of success in pharmaceutical education, but the basis for success in life.[10]

Though a partial motivation for the inclusion of liberal studies may have been to supply a "finishing school" process for instilling social graces or as a passport for entry into a more prestigious social class,[11] there was also an early recognition of the transformative role of liberal education to prepare graduates to analyze, synthesize, and solve problems:

> This, however, unquestionably is true, that he who has at least a glimpse of how the present has evolved out of the past will be less dogmatic for such historic information and will be in a better position to recognize the possibilities of the future; that he who has become acquainted with the scientific method will waste less time in solving problems of everyday professional life than he who merely learned to do things according to a rule of thumb. ...Let me therefore make an earnest plea for the cultivation of the cultural phases of the pharmaceutical courses of study as opposed to the more apparent technical phases.[12]

Implicit in this recommendation is the understanding that general education should not be simply added on to a professional program but should be co-extensive with it. Similarly, current recommendations are not to design a curriculum in which general action is merely a prelude to professional education but is integrated with it. The Professional Preparation Network had concluded:

> Based on our experiences, we view current efforts toward higher education reform as incomplete, because they fail to stress the responsibility of educators to increase the integration of liberal and professional study.[13]

In pharmacy, the AACP Focus Group on Liberalization of the Profession agreed:

> Education in the liberal arts can and should provide an important base of perspectives and intellectual skills necessary for the development and growth of professionals. A primary goal

of colleges of pharmacy should be the development of strategies for integrating and building upon these perspectives and skills from the liberal arts within the professional education of each pharmacy student.[14]

Still, the strategies to accomplish this integration or even a clear understanding of what it means has remained somewhat elusive.[15] "Liberalization of the professional curriculum," for instance, is commonly misunderstood. "Liberalization" in this context is not shorthand for the liberal arts or a humanistic body of knowledge; it does not mean working Shakespeare into therapeutics or art history into a medicinal chemistry course. The Professional Preparation Network explicitly rejected the notions that adding more liberal arts courses to the professional curriculum or offering liberal arts courses parallel with professional courses is the optimum solution for integrating professional and liberal education.[16] Rather, liberalization of the professional curriculum means bringing to the professional courses a set of attitudes, habits, values, skills, and teaching practices that traditionally have been associated with liberal education—both humanistic and scientific.

Some clarification is provided by the American Association of Colleges and Universities (AAC&U) Project on Accreditation and Assessment, which in 2004 reaffirmed this re-visioning of professional education:

> In this project, leaders from the agencies accrediting professional programs were unanimous in declaring a liberal education is not impractical or an unnecessary luxury; rather, it is essential to professional success in their fields. …a high quality program should integrate liberal and professional education.[17]

The educational plan should be not to teach the abilities in succession, with general education relegated to preprofessional study and professional abilities following later in the curriculum. Nor should the plan be to teach the two sets of abilities in parallel but separate and distinct courses. The goal is to integrate the learning of general and professional abilities, for the professional abilities build upon the general. Thinking, communicating, and ethical decision making, for instance, are components of many professional abilities, such as recommending drug therapy or educating health care professionals. Once instructors recognize that the professional ability outcomes are combinations of general abilities, they can develop a number of innovative teaching strategies that allow students to practice general abilities within professional contexts.

In other words, general education need not be entirely content-specific or discipline-specific. In one sense, it is a matter of how the material is taught, not what is taught.

> General education is to be had … anywhere in the college curriculum, whether the discipline in question is traditionally liberal or frankly professional—as long as the instructor plans carefully not just the substantive information she is imparting, but the qualities of complex reasoning, and the subtle contexts of culture and value, that she is also presenting.[18]

For instance, an instructor in a course on herbal products can lecture on toxicity, side-effects, drug interactions, efficacy, mechanisms of action, etc. so that students leave the class informed about facts surrounding herbals. But the instructor can also use herbal products content as a vehicle to develop students' thinking, communication, and ethical decision making (general ability outcomes) as they relate to counseling patients regarding the use and abuse of herbal products (a professional ability).[19] In the process, students of course still learn about classifications, structures, uses, efficacy, safety, etc., but they also learn to analyze and evaluate claims made about herbal products, communicate information about herbals to targeted audiences, and to recognize and reconcile ethical dilemmas in the marketing and use of herbal products. To develop such general and professional abilities, though, students must practice them. That means, the course must be transformed from a lecture-based, content-centered approach to an active-learning, ability-based approach in which students practice the abilities in class or in assignments such as analyzing herbal products literature and advertising, comparing different responses given by online pharmacies to questions regarding the use of herbal products, writing simulated responses to online pharmacy questions that raise safety issues, and solving cases that present ethical conflicts regarding the recommendation and use of herbal products. It is in such practice, when guided by clear performance criteria and specific assessment feedback, that students develop both general and professional ability outcomes.[20]

> Education in the liberal arts can and should provide an important base of perspectives and intellectual skills necessary for the development and growth of professionals. A primary goal of colleges of pharmacy should be the development of strategies for integrating and building upon these perspectives and skills from the liberal arts within the professional education of each pharmacy student.
>
> *AACP Focus Group on Liberalization of the Profession*

What is being proposed, then, by an integration of general and professional ability outcomes is not so much the inclusion of a new, intrusive body of knowledge but a different orientation within professional education. Professional education without the general abilities tends toward training and application. Professional abilities are the context in which students develop critical thinking, communication, ethical decision-making.

As we shall see, problem-based learning, case studies, simulations, active learning, early experiential activities, service learning, assessment as learning, and ability-based assessment are among the educational strategies faculty are using to develop general abilities within profession contexts, helping students to extending themselves beyond technical competence. But there is a deeper connection still between professional and general learning.

Doing and Being in Pharmacy Education

Professional education and general education are more intimately intertwined beyond the fact that they seek to develop common intellectual skills. That connection, again, is rooted in the nature of a profession.

Despite some alarming current trends in a number of professions, professionals do not have "customers"; they have "clients," "patients," "students." As we have seen, the professional's relationship to the person is not mercantile but fiduciary. A professional has special knowledge that he or she uses to touch the life of a person so intimately that that person must have complete trust, complete faith, in the professional; the client/patient must believe the professional will act in his or her best interest, not self-interest.

Pharmacy's long-standing association with a product has obscured for some that pharmacy is not an occupation (based on mercantile relationships) but a profession (based on fiduciary relationships). As pharmaceutical care has become more entrenched as the philosophy of pharmacy practice, it is clearer what a radical change in perspective is needed regarding pharmacists' responsibilities. William Zellmer astutely observes:

> I think we have greatly underestimated the magnitude of the paradigm shift that pharmaceutical care embodies. ...Let me remind you of Thomas Moore's definition of soul: "It has to do with depth, value, relatedness, heart, and personal substance." People want and need pharmacists with those characteristics—pharmacists with soul. Let's dedicate ourselves to remaking this occupation of ours into a profession that gives people what they want and need.[21]

Pharmaceutical care as a mission for pharmacy practice brings into high relief the responsibilities of pharmacy professionals: "Professions exist to serve society." "[Pharmaceutical care] advocates a covenantal relationship between pharmacy practitioners and patients. ..." "Pharmaceutical care focuses pharmacists' attitudes, behaviors, commitments, concerns, ethics, functions, knowledge, responsibilities, and skills on the provision of drug therapy..."[22]

What are the implications for pharmacy education? The answer is obvious: "Pharmaceutical education inculcates students with the values necessary to serve society as caring, ethical, learning professionals and enlightened citizens."[23] A more difficult question is, what are we doing in our colleges of pharmacy to accomplish this task?

This connects to general education in two ways. First, the integration of general and professional abilities. An ability, unlike a skill or an objective, is itself a combination of knowledge, skills, attitudes, values, dispositions, motivations, and habits. Most often in the classroom, however, it is the knowledge that is prioritized, and to some extent so are skills, particularly in labs and clinical experiences. Less conscious attention is applied to attitudes, motivations, dispositions, values, and habits. In the general ability of communication, which is of course related to the professional ability of patient counseling, empathy and caring may be just as important as knowledge of drugs and disease states in order to ensure patient compliance. Identifying the components of each ability outcome—the knowledge, skills, and attitudinal components—can prompt instructors to ask, "What in my course is done to develop each of these components?" and, more importantly, "What can I do to make sure that students in my class have opportunities to practice and reflect upon abilities that integrate knowing, doing, and evaluating?" Preparing students to achieve the ability to "provide patient-centered care" demands innovative instructional approaches when it is acknowledged that components of such an ability include:

- Take into account patients' individuality, emotional needs, values, and life issues.
- Provide care for patients in the context of the culture, heath status, and health needs of the population of which each is a member.
- Provide care that reflects the whole person.[24]

Second, professional education, like liberal education, ideally prepares graduates not just for doing but also for being. Professional education not only trains pharmacists but also educates persons who are pharmacists. Despite the skeptics, such dimensions as character, service, citizenship, and caring can be "taught." Not taught in didactic fashion and then tested through an exam, of course. But these dimensions can be promoted and developed by challenging students with value frameworks, providing opportunities to kindle their sometimes latent desires to care and serve, scheduling time for structured reflection, and giving formative feedback to help them to grow.[25]

> General education is to be had ... anywhere in the college curriculum, whether the discipline in question is traditionally liberal or frankly professional—as long as the instructor plans carefully not just the substantive information she is imparting, but the qualities of complex reasoning, and the subtle contexts of culture and value, that she is also presenting.
>
> *Linda Salamon*

In class work and experiential programs, faculty can thematize service, care, and fiduciary responsibilities. Probably every discipline from biology through pharmacotherapy can stimulate growth in self-awareness and the development of a world view. Some pharmacy faculty try to stimulate students to connect content to broader life issues by incorporating literature, art, or film into the courses. For example, instructors dealing with patient compliance and issues of cultural diversity might supplement their lectures with Anne Fadiman's book The Spirit Catches You and You Fall Down, which documents the failure of the American medical system to deal effectively with the epilepsy of a young Hmong child.[26] The goal of such assignments is not simply to develop better people but to ensure better health care. Particularly at an advantage are those pharmacy institutions that allow collaboration with general education faculty to develop the type of general education program that will support these professional goals of character, service, citizenship, and caring—not just in the general education courses but also in the professional courses. Encouraging is the number of pharmacy schools that have adopted service learning. When students provide service to people in need and are encouraged to reflect upon their experiences within a structured program, they tend to grow in character and attitude.[27] And, of course, it is impossible to overestimate the value and effectiveness of modeling.

There is a larger picture. The benefits of distance education are extremely promising, and more innovations should be encouraged. But it should be recognized that distance learning alone does not provide a college education. Part of a college education, in fact much of it, occurs outside of the classroom, in the college setting and its co-curricular programs. This is especially true in the development of students' attitudes and character. Effective development of students' character and attitudes lies not simply with the curriculum but with co-curricular programs and the culture of the college. It may be true in pharmacy as in medicine,

> ...that although matters of technical information and the transmission of technical skills traditionally have been thought to lie at the heart of the medical educational system, medical training at root is a process of moral enculturation, and that in transmitting normative rules regarding behavior and emotions to its trainees, the medical school functions as a moral community. ...Formal instruction in ethics makes only a small contribution to that community. ...An entire curriculum will not decisively reshape a student's personality or ensure ethical conduct in the future.[28]

Attitude, values, and character are critical in the teaching of professional ability outcomes. One researcher concludes that in the solution of bioethical problems, for instance, "The cultivation of a morally sensitive, caring, and compassionate character probably counts for more in the end than ... analytical skills."[29] Undoubtedly the same is true of other professional abilities. Students who are committed, empathic, ethical, and caring will become better providers of pharmaceutical care. Needed are models in pharmacy education in which the enculturation of professional values and the development of character occur in premeditated rather than haphazard fashion within classrooms, experiential settings, and campus life.

Guideposts for Integration

Two recent works provide guideposts toward greater integration of liberal and professional education.

Often liberal arts is perceived as an enrichment of professional education. Lee Shulman in "Professing the Liberal Arts" proposes the reverse.[30] Shulman identifies three deficiencies of liberal education: "amnesia" (I forgot it); illusion of learning (I never knew it); and inert ideas (I don't know what to do with it). He sees a revitalization of the liberal arts through professional education because inherent in professional education are the principles that can help to overcome amnesia, illusory understanding, and inert ideas:

Activity	doing things with learning
Reflection	thinking about what you are doing
Collaboration	learning with others and reciprocal teaching
Passion	emotional involvement through connecting what you are doing to present and future goals
Community	an institutional structure that nourishes such learning

Noting that the goal of a profession is service, Shulman links professional education not only to technical competence but also to character development: "The professional educator's challenge is to help future professors develop and shape a robust moral vision that will guide their practice and provide a prism of justice and virtue through which to reflect on their actions."

Another beacon is *Learning that Lasts: Integrating Learning, Development, and Performance in College and Beyond*, by Marcia Mentkowski and associates from Alverno College.[31] This book promotes a restructuring of undergraduate education in such a way that liberal arts, professional education, and development of moral character are integrated within a carefully constructed college experience. The authors describe the efforts of Alverno College and of various consortia to connect learning, work, personal life, and citizenship,

> The professional educator's challenge is to help future professors develop and shape a robust moral vision that will guide their practice and provide a prism of justice and virtue through which to reflect on their actions.
>
> *Lee Shulman*

concluding that a college's curricular and co-curricular programs can help students to integrate learning, development as a person, and effective performance in the workplace, family, and community. Once again, the focus is on how professional and general education complement one another:

> We found that professional performance is connected to the liberal arts and its values traditions; each of the ability factors reflected a particular integration of liberal learning and professional abilities. (185)

> We found that students first came to appreciate liberal learning as they connected it to expanded understanding of professional role identities, laying a foundation for their development of a sense of purpose. The liberal arts exerted a long-lasting influence on the integration of the persons, and the way the individual enacts values of compassion, collaboration, continued learning, open-mindedness, and integrity. (203)

The key is to create and continually refine a learning program that centers on the student's continuing growth in abilities, perspectives, commitments, and moral judgments. Learning that Lasts describes the processes and results of over 20 years of experience in developing such a program.

It may well be that when pharmacy educators call for an integration of general and professional education, they are talking about eliciting durable learning, learning that lasts. That is, according to the findings at Alverno, learning that is integrative, experiential, self-aware and reflective, self-assessed and self-regarding, developmental and individual, transitional and transformative, active and interactive, independent and collaborative, situated and transferable, deep and expansive, purposeful and responsible.

> We found that professional performance is connected to the liberal arts and its values traditions; each of the ability factors reflected a particular integration of liberal learning and professional abilities.
>
> *Marcia Mentkowski*

This is an ambitious project, extending far beyond tinkering with the curriculum or adding active learning experiences within courses. However, with its emphasis on doing what one knows and on developing the student as a learner, person, citizen, and professional, such a program can produce deep, durable, meaningful learning, the type of learning that pharmacy education has set as a goal over the past 15 years.

Summary

So, what does the integration of general and professional ability outcomes mean? It means teaching general and professional abilities in the same courses in both the preprofessional and professional years, adopting the explicit goal of helping students to improve as problem-solvers, critical thinkers, ethical decision-makers, and communicators within the discipline taught in the course. It means moving beyond content (not away from content) toward a student-centered pedagogy that stresses active and lifelong learning. In

Shulman's terms, it means creating educational experiences that combine activity, reflection, collaboration, passion, and community.

It means focusing explicitly on developing and espousing curricular and co-curricular programs that promote the values and character of individuals who will honor their professional duty to abide by fiduciary relationships for the people they serve, people they not only care for but care about.[32]

It means creating an academic community dedicated to learning that lasts, integrative, experiential, self-reflective, purposeful, active, transformative learning which prepares graduates for success in the workplace, family, and community.

Over the past 20 years pharmacy educators have made tremendous strides in developing innovative curricula that incorporate the principles of active, student-centered learning, problem-based learning, service learning, and ability-based education. A continuing conscious effort to integrate general and professional ability outcomes might provide a tighter framework for organizing educational programs that enable graduates to perform effectively as professionals, citizens, and family members.

Questions for Reflection

1. Which more informs your own teaching orientation and practice—a teaching paradigm or a learning paradigm? Can you cite examples?
2. In your teaching, what emphasis do you place on training and what emphasis on education?
3. To what extent are general ability outcomes integrated into your teaching? In what ways could they be?
4. Is it really a possibility for pharmacy education to be "transformative" in the sense discussed in this chapter? What can you do in your own teaching to promote "learning that lasts"?

Notes

1. Joint Commission of Pharmacy Practitioners. Future vision of pharmacy practice. In Maine LL. The class of 2015. Am J Pharm Educ 2005;69(3):article 56.
2. Institute of Medicine. To err is human: building a safer health system. Washington DC: The National Academy Press, 2001. See also, Institute of Medicine. Crossing the quality chasm: a new health system for the 21st century. Washington DC: The National Academy Press, 2001.
3. Institute of Medicine. Greiner AC, Knebel E, eds. Health professions education: a bridge to quality. Washington DC: The National Academies Press, 2003:1-3. The IOM competencies were one resource used in the reformulation of the 2004 CAPE Educational Outcomes prepared by the American Association of Colleges of Pharmacy.
4. Barr RB, Tagg J. From teaching to learning: a new paradigm for undergraduate education. Change 1995;27:12-25.
5. Of course, the situation is much more complex than this schema implies. For a discussion of learning theory, see Donovan MS, Bransford JD, Pellegrino JW, eds. How people learn: bridging research and practice. Washington DC: National Academy Press, 1999. Kolb D.A. Experiential learning: experience as the source of learning and development. Englewood Cliffs,

NJ: Prentice Hall, 1984. Gardner H. Multiple intelligences: the theory in practice. New York: Basic Books, 1999. Gardner H. Intelligence reframed: multiple intelligence for the 21st century. New York: Basic Books; 1999. Armstrong T. Multiple intelligences in the classroom. Alexandria, VA: Association for Supervision and Curriculum Development, 1994. Belenky M, Clinchy B, Goldberger NR, Tarule JM. Women's ways of knowing: the development of self, voice and mind. New York: Basic Books, 1986. Studies within pharmacy include, Shuck AA, Phillips CR. Assessing pharmacy students' learning styles and personality types: A ten-year analysis. Am J Pharm Educ 1999; 63: 27-33. Pungente MD, Wasan KM, Moffett C. Using learning styles to evaluate first-year pharmacy students' preferences toward different activities associated with the problem-based learning approach. Am J of Pharm Educ 2003;66:119-24; Austin Z. Development and validation of the pharmacists' inventory of learning styles (PILS). Am J Pharm Educ 2004;68:article 37.

6. Cohen JL. Chair report for the Academic Affairs Committee. Am J Pharm Educ 1988;52:409-11.

7. American Association of Colleges of Pharmacy. Educational outcomes. Center for the Advancement of Pharmaceutical Education (CAPE). Alexandria, VA: American Association of Colleges of Pharmacy, 1994.

8. American Association of Colleges of Pharmacy. Educational outcomes. Center for the Advancement of Pharmaceutical Education (CAPE). Alexandria, VA: American Association of Colleges of Pharmacy 2004.

9. See Maine LL. CAPE outcomes 2004: What do pharmacists do? Am J Pharm Educ 2004; 68(3):article 78.

10. Quoted in Newcomer J, Bunnell KP, McGrath EJ. Liberal education and pharmacy. New York: Institute of Higher Education, Columbia University, 1960.

11. Parrish E. Proceedings of the American Pharmaceutical Association at the Twentieth Annual Meeting, 1872 In Newcomer J, Bunnell KP, McGrath EJ. Liberal education and pharmacy. New York: Institute of Higher Education, Teachers College, Columbia University, 1960:23.

12. Kremers E. Proceedings of the American Conference of Pharmaceutical Faculties at the Fourth Annual Meeting, 1903. Cited in Newcomer J, Bunnell KP, McGrath EJ. Liberal education and pharmacy. New York: Institute of Higher Education, Columbia University, 1960:25.

13. Stark JS, Lowther MA. Strengthening the ties that bind: integrating undergraduate liberal and professional study. The Professional Preparation Network, Ann Arbor, MI: University of Michigan, 1988.

14. Chalmers RK, Grotpeter JJ, et al. Ability-based outcome goals for the professional curriculum: a report of the Focus Group on Liberalization of the Professional Curriculum. Am J Pharm Educ 1992;56:304-9.

15. For a summary, see Zlatic TD. Integrating education: chair report of the 1999/2000 Academic Affairs Committee, American Association of Colleges of Pharmacy. Am J Pharm Educ 2000;64:8S-15S

16. Stark JS, Lowther MA. Strengthening the ties that bind: integrating undergraduate liberal and professional study. The Professional Preparation Network. Ann Arbor, MI: University of Michigan, 1988:9.

17. Taking responsibility for the quality of the baccalaureate degree: a report from the greater expectations project on accreditation and assessment. Washington DC: American Association of Colleges and Universities, 2004: iv.

18. Salamon LB. Integrity in the pharmacy curriculum. Am J Pharm Educ 1985;49:361-5.
19. Zlatic TD, Nowak DM, Sylvester D. Integrating general and professional education through a study of herbal products: an intercollegiate collaboration. Am J Pharm Educ 2000;64:83-94.
20. See Ability-based learning programs. Rev ed. Milwaukee, WI: Alverno Institute, 1994. Also see Chapter 6 of this book.7
21. Zellmer WA. Searching for the soul of pharmacy. Am J Health Syst Pharm 1996;53:1911-6. For a discussion of the importance of relationships in pharmacy practice and an application to pharmacy of Martin Buber's analysis of "I-Thou" and "I-It" orientations, see Berger BA. Communication skills for pharmacists: building relationships, improving care. 2nd ed. Washington DC: American Pharmacists Association, 2005.
22. American Association of Colleges of Pharmacy. Background paper I: what is the mission of pharmaceutical education? [1990]. Am J Pharm Educ 1993;57:374-6.
23. Ibid.
24. Institute of Medicine. Greiner AC, Knebel E, eds. Health professions education: a bridge to quality. Washington DC: The National Academies Press, 2003:53.
25. Spiro H. What is empathy and can it be taught? Ann Intern Med 1992;116:843-6.
26. Fadiman A. The spirit catches you and you fall down: a Hmong child, her American doctors, and the collision of two cultures. New York: Farrar, Straus, and Giroux, 1997.
27. Nickman NA. (Re-)learning to care: use of service-learning as an early professionalization experience. Am J Pharm Educ 1998;62:380-7. Murawski MM, Muraski D, Wilson M. Service-learning and pharmaceutical education: an exploratory survey. Am J Pharm Educ 1999;63:160-4. Piper B, DeYoung M, Lamsam G. Student perceptions of a service-learning experience. Am J Pharm Educ 2000;64:159-65.
28. Hafferty FW, Franks R. The hidden curriculum, ethics teaching, and the structure of medical education. Acad Med 1994;69:861-71.
29. Holmes RL. The limited relevance of analytical ethics to the problems of bioethics. The J Med Philos 1990;15:143-59.
30. Shulman LS. Professing the liberal arts. In Orrill R, ed. Education and democracy: re-imagining liberal learning in America. New York: The College Board, 1997.
31. Mentkowski M and Associates. Learning that lasts: integrating learning, development, and performance in college and beyond. San Francisco: Jossey-Bass, 2000.
32. Reich WT. What care can mean for pharmaceutical ethics. Journal of Pharmacy Teaching, 1996;5:1-17.

Chapter 3: Defining Critical Thinking within Professional Contexts

In its 1985 seminal report, Integrity in the College Curriculum, the American Association of Colleges (AAC) insisted on inquiry, abstract logical thinking, and critical analysis as essential minimum components of any college curriculum.[1] Soon thereafter this AAC report was endorsed by the American Association of Colleges of Pharmacy (AACP),[2] which recognized a need for graduates to become effective thinkers and communicators within the profession of pharmacy,[3] this during a time when there was concern about "the increasing reliance on the didactic format as a means of presenting coursework, which leads to a one-way exchange of information technical school environment where facts, but not ideas and values, get transferred to our students."[4]

AACP's Commission to Implement Change in Pharmaceutical Education clearly pointed out one direction that needed to be taken:

> Of special significance for pharmaceutical education is the question of how critical thinking is taught and evaluated. …Although critical thinking is a universally desired educational outcome, professionals particularly need a repertoire of thinking strategies that will enable them to acquire, evaluate and synthesize information and knowledge. …Critical thinking fosters a questioning attitude among professionals; and it is a prerequisite skill in making judgments.[5]

Since the early 1990s, this challenge has been met by a number of innovative pharmacy educators who have implemented strategies for the teaching and evaluation of critical thinking. Subsequent research has corroborated that there is in fact a connection between critical thinking[6] and success in pharmacy school: "Critical thinking skills are predictive of student performance in clerkships and pharmacy practice courses."[7]

Nonetheless, integrating critical thinking into a professional program can be fraught with difficulties. "Critical thinking" itself is a slippery term. First of all, critical thinking is not some "thing." Thinking is an activity. When we give names to activities, we sometimes pretend we are dealing with substances frozen in space and time for easy inspection. For instance, thunder is an event, not a thing; silence is what happens when the event stops. Thinking, too, whether critical or not, is an event. It is not something we can put under a microscope or subject to spectral analysis. It is not something that stands still or stays the same. And the fact that it takes place internally means that much of our knowledge about thinking is inferential, although medical technology is making remarkable strides in helping us to picture brain activity.

Commission to Implement Change in Pharmaceutical Education

Second, critical thinking is not one activity but a series of mental processes, a complex integration of multiple abilities that finds different expression in different circumstances and in different people. Names try to capture these processes and make them discrete, but in reality the processes blend and merge in a number of ways that are beyond our current understanding. In our taxonomies we can conceptually separate analysis from evaluation or tease out creativity from problem solving, but seldom in practice do we make such neat distinctions. Cognitive science warns us about being reductive in our study of thinking; not one but multiple intelligences help us to respond to the complexities of our world.

> The new mission of pharmacy practice is pharmaceutical care. Pharmaceutical care serves as the basis for strategic planning regarding the depth, curricular outcomes, content, and educational processes of pharmacy education.
>
> *Commission to Implement Change in Pharmaceutical Education*

Third, "critical thinking" is pursued differently in different contexts. In academia, where critical thinking is most explicitly taught, such contexts are called disciplines. At theoretical levels, psychologists, philosophers, and physicists will debate the real definition of critical thinking. At practical levels students moving through a curriculum encounter these multiple contexts and become confused. Craig Nelson from the University of Indiana points out that analysis, for instance, means something entirely different in biology than in literature class. Bright students who do exceptionally well in one discipline may do poorly in the other because they have not learned the differences. The biology major who has been trained to use analysis as a taxonomic process will experience grief if she attempts to apply the same skill to a literature assignment that asks her to exercise analytical skills when comparing King Lear and Macbeth.

For some skeptics already overburdened with teaching and pressured by research, the complexity and lack of concreteness are enough to dismiss critical thinking as another pedagogical buzz word that, if we stall long enough, will pass out of existence before we must deal with it. That is a possibility but, if the last 2,500 years are any indication, it is not likely. As protean and amorphous as it may appear to be, critical thinking deserves some attention from educators, including pharmacy educators.

For instance, do you agree that the following three paragraphs reveal different types of thinking:

(1) Late at night I lie awake remembering the last time I saw Elvis in concert and thinking about what I will say to him when I corner him outside of the Iowa City delicatessen that the National Enquirer says he visits every Thursday. I try to imagine what he will be wearing and how he will respond when I tell him I have memorized the lyrics of every song he ever sang. I picture the look on Mary Jane's face when I tell her about how we spent the evening together.

(2) I systematically have gathered and studied all available reports on the sightings of Elvis and have calculated that 75% of the time Elvis is seen east of the Mississippi and 52% of the time he is seen after 4:00 in the afternoon. I am able to determine my chances of seeing him in St. Louis at 10:00 in the morning are a very slim 18%; the best place to meet him is in New York after dark. Though I have very little money, by carefully coordinating with five car transport companies I am able to get to New York for free, and to support myself while waiting for Elvis I get a job selling foot-long weenies on Fifth Avenue from 3:00 to 9:00 each evening.

(3) Since 1957 I have been a fan of Elvis and have desperately hoped that the "King" is still alive, hiding out so he can lead a peaceful life. However, the only places that I read about Elvis being spotted are in the grocery tabloids, never in the *New York Times* or in the local paper. As much as I would like it to be true, I must conclude that the latest report about Elvis being seen with Michael Landon at an all-night poodle-grooming salon in Vermont is probably simply another hoax.

The first person is highly imaginative, perhaps creative, but his imagination is never far from the world of dreams. He obviously is thinking but is he thinking well? Within the framework of her beliefs, the second person is an extremely logical and creative problem-solver, but like other fanatics (e.g., astrologers, cultists, conspiracy theorists) her problem-solving, as comprehensive and complex as it may be, makes sense only within the circumscribed world in which she lives; she never questions the framework within which she operates to determine if it is attached to anything real. The third thinker seems to demonstrate a willingness and ability to weigh evidence and make appropriate judgments in spite of his emotional drive to believe the contrary. It is this last type of thinking that might be labeled "critical."

As we shall see, clustered around critical thinking are such phrases and concepts as metacognition; awareness, critique, and correction of our thinking processes; thinking about thinking so as to improve our thinking; recognition of our own assumptions and uncovering assumptions in others' arguments; probing the reasons for our beliefs; recognizing logical errors; understanding why some arguments for belief are better than others; establishing and evaluating criteria; decision making; problem solving. Skills that are common to many definitions of critical thinking are analysis, synthesis, and evaluation. Critical thinking abilities integrate skills with knowledge, skills, attitudes, habits, dispositions, and values; there are affective and ethical as well as cognitive components to critical thinking. The following pages attempt to provide background about such concepts so that pharmacy faculty can examine the content and goals of their courses and rotations. The two goals are:

1. Determine your purposes and course outcomes regarding thinking.
2. Review the critical thinking literature to determine what models or concepts can facilitate your teaching of thinking skills.

Subsequent chapters provide background for planning course activities and assignments that stimulate thinking, and for making assessment of thinking skills part of the learning process.

Determining Course Purpose and Outcomes

Although some pharmacy faculty may not have extensive background in critical thinking instruction, they do have ideas about what their students must be able to do to practice pharmaceutical care in the next decades.

Critical thinking instruction should build upon that knowledge. Faculty should begin inductively with an inventory of their own courses in light of what they want their students to be able to know and do. That way, critical thinking instruction can grow organically out of the discipline; it will be integrated into the course rather than grafted onto it. Later, faculty can review the literature to find concepts, theories, and models that will help them to expand, refine, and develop the thinking skills they would like their students to learn. Reflect on the following questions:

1. What is the purpose(s) of my course/rotation within the curriculum?
2. Am I satisfied with how well my course/rotation is meeting that purpose(s)?
3. What evidence do I have that my course/rotation is successful/not successful?
4. What do I want my students to know when they finish my course/rotation? (Be explicit but do not simply itemize facts.)
5. What do I want my students to be able to do with what they will know when they finish my course/rotation? (Be explicit.)
6. What thinking abilities and skills must the students develop in order to achieve the outcomes expected of them in this course/rotation?

Answers to these questions are the beginning of an iterative process. Once instructors have made an initial attempt to define what they want to accomplish in terms of higher order thinking, they can then review the critical thinking literature to determine what definitions and tools best suit their goals. Then, the literature review might prompt a reformulation of what can and should be accomplished in terms of higher order thinking in pharmacy courses and experiential programs.

Defining Critical Thinking

The tasks of defining critical thinking and creating a program for critical thinking instruction must be themselves a practice of critical thinking. The process must be not simple application but also analysis, synthesis, and judgment.

Thinking skill instruction should be developed out of the desired outcomes and the subject matter of the course. Faculty should be responsible for determining and defining what thinking skills their students need. However, that determination and definition should not occur in a vacuum or solipsistic reverie. The faculty's plans should be informed by an analysis and synthesis of what researchers have discovered and conjectured about thinking abilities and pedagogy.

Faculty wanting to create a plan for incorporating critical thinking into their teaching can encounter a similar problem facing pharmacy students: there is too much content to process. The Educational Resources Information Center (ERIC) database of educational references currently lists approximately 11,709 citations to critical thinking in the literature of multiple disciplines!

To provide an entrée into the scholarship of critical thinking, what follows is a limited and somewhat arbitrary literature review of critical thinking. Not everything in this survey will be pertinent to your teaching goals. Feel free to pass quickly over sections that are not relevant to your goals. As you read this survey, mark sections that help you to answer the following questions:

1. What definition(s) of higher order thinking skills can best facilitate my course preparation and teaching of critical thinking?
2. What model(s) of higher order thinking skills can best facilitate my course preparation and teaching of critical thinking?
3. What discrete thinking skills are most important for my course/rotation?

Definitions and Models of Critical Thinking

Entering the world of critical thinking literature is a little bit like entering *Alice's Adventures in Wonderland*:

> "'But 'glory' doesn't mean 'a nice knockdown argument,'" Alice objected.
> "When I use a word," Humpty Dumpty said, in a rather scornful tone, "it means just what I choose it to mean—neither more nor less."
> "The question is," said Alice, "whether you can make words mean so many different things."
> "The question is," said Humpty Dumpty, "which is to be master—that's all."

The term "critical thinking" likewise serves a number of masters. Among the discourses that have appropriated the term are philosophy and logic, psychology and cognitive science, education, the sciences, and social theory (e.g., post-structuralism, feminism). Sometimes the term's boundaries are expanded to include other terms such as higher order thinking, creativity, problem solving, decision making, and metacognition.

Popularly the words "critical thinking" are used loosely as a catch-phrase for a wide array of thinking skills that are necessary for political freedom and technological superiority in an increasingly complex world. In this loose sense, critical thinking can best be defined by what it is not. When educational reformers, government officials, and business leaders sound the alarm about the need for critical thinking in school curricula, they are concerned about such practices as rote memorization, passive learning, decontextualized learning experiences, and objective testing. "Critical thinking" becomes the generic buzz words to denote the alternatives to what are regarded as inadequate educational practices.

Within academic disciplines, critical thinking takes on stricter definitions, but naturally the disciplines' differing paradigms, methodologies, and taxonomies prevent a univocal definition. And, of course, within the same disciplines are a number of schools and individuals who define critical thinking differently.

Informal Logic and Argument

Critical thinking has a firm foundation within the philosophical tradition. Socrates is often cited as the first great paragon of critical thinking: a person who was not satisfied with appearances, who continually probed and asked embarrassing questions, who examined thinking to ferret out indefensible assumptions and unwarranted conclusions. In this definition, the critical thinker gives reasons for beliefs, understands the criteria for

Richard Paul's 35 Dimensions of Critical Thought

A. Affective Strategies

S-1 thinking independently
S-2 developing insight into egocentricity or sociocentricity
S-3 exercising fair-mindedness
S-4 exploring thoughts underlying feelings and feelings underlying thoughts
S-5 developing intellectual humility and suspending judgment
S-6 developing intellectual courage
S-7 developing intellectual good faith or integrity
S-8 developing intellectual perseverance
S-9 developing confidence in reason

B. Cognitive Strategies—Macro-Abilities

S-10 refining generalizations and avoiding oversimplifications
S-11 comparing analogous situations: transferring insights to new contexts
S-12 developing one's perspective: creating or exploring beliefs, arguments, or theories
S-13 clarifying issues, conclusions, or beliefs
S-14 clarifying and analyzing the meanings of works or phrases
S-15 developing criteria for evaluation: clarifying values and standards
S-16 evaluating the credibility of sources of information
S-17 questioning deeply: raising and pursuing root or significant questions
S-18 analyzing or evaluating arguments, interpretations, beliefs, or theories
S-19 generating or assessing solutions
S-20 analyzing or evaluating actions or policies
S-21 reading critically: clarifying or critiquing texts
S-22 listening critically: the art of silent dialogue
S-23 making interdisciplinary connections
S-24 practicing Socratic discussion: clarifying and questioning beliefs, theories, or perspectives
S-25 reasoning dialogically: comparing perspectives, interpretations, or theories
S-26 reasoning dialectically: evaluating perspectives, interpretations, or theories

C. Cognitive Strategies—Micro-Skills

S-27 comparing and contrasting ideals with actual practice
S-28 thinking precisely about thinking: using critical vocabulary
S-29 noting significant similarities and differences
S-30 examining or evaluating assumptions
S-31 distinguishing relevant from irrelevant facts
S-32 making plausible inferences, predictions, or interpretations
S-33 giving reasons and evaluating evidence and alleged facts
S-34 recognizing contradictions
S-35 exploring implications and consequences

Reprinted with permission of the Foundation for Critical Thinking and Moral Critique, *www.criticalthinking.org*. Center for Critical Thinking and Moral Critique, Sonoma State University, Rohnert Park, CA; 1990.

some arguments being better than others, defends beliefs in a logical manner, and is open to modifying beliefs in face of compelling contrary evidence.

Richard Paul from the Center for Critical Thinking and Moral Critique at Sonoma State University in California represents this tradition. Critical thinking is an "interlocking complex of skills, attitudes, passions . ... not exactly a species of thinking; rather, it is a species of living. It is living, in Socrates' phrase, an examined life, a *deeply* examined life." Paul identifies 35 dimensions of critical thinking and divides them into three categories: Affective Strategies (e.g., thinking independently, developing intellectual courage); Macro-Ability Cognitive Strategies (e.g., clarifying issues, developing criteria for evaluation, reasoning dialectically); and Micro-Skills Cognitive Strategies (e.g., examining assumptions, exploring implications). Paul dismisses critical thinking theories that attempt to be value-neutral. Implicit in his definition of critical thinking in what he calls the "strong sense" are values and even morals; the critical thinker must grow out of ego- and socio-centricity as he or she develops skills such as logical analysis and attitudes such as fair-mindedness and perseverance.[8]

In the late 1980s, 46 people from multiple disciplines (52% were from philosophy) assembled to form an interactive panel of critical thinking experts using the Delphi Method.[9] They came to a consensus that the following are critical thinking cognitive skills: interpretation, analysis, evaluation, inference, explanation, self-regulation. In addition, they agreed on 19 affective dispositions of critical thinking, including inquisitiveness, confidence in one's own reasoning, open and fair-mindedness, as well as willingness to modify beliefs. In its 12 recommendations regarding the definition, teaching, and assessment of critical thinking, the panel emphasized a need for a holistic conception of critical thinking that integrates critical thinking cognitive skills and affective dispositions. A liberal arts education and modeling of critical thinking by instructors are seen as extremely effective methods for teaching critical thinking. Peter Facione, the Delphi Report writer, developed the California Critical Thinking Test and the California Critical Thinking Dispositions Test to measure student development in both the cognitive and affective realms of critical thinking.

Influenced by Robert Ennis' definition of critical thinking as "reasonable, reflective thinking that is focused on deciding what to believe or do," early attempts at defining critical thinking stressed formal and informal reasoning and the logical analysis of arguments.[10] This led to a wave of stand-alone critical thinking courses that taught no content other than general thinking skills; the assumption was that students could transfer the general skills to the academic disciplines.

John McPeck and others eventually countered that analysis of argument constitutes a relatively small portion of critical thinking. Instead, McPeck defined critical thinking as the "reflective use of skepticism within the problem area under consideration" or "the propensity and skill to engage in an activity with reflective skepticism."[11] The implications of this are that students cannot become effective critical thinkers without sufficient knowledge about what they are thinking, and it is unlikely that general thinking skills can be learned that will help the student become a more effective thinker within the academic disciplines. Critical thinking must be learned within contexts and must entail knowledge of facts, rules, and processes within those contexts. But McPeck, too, concludes that a liberal education has not yet been surpassed as a method for teaching critical thinking.[12] For development of critical thinking in such an education, instructors must encourage students to recognize that the facts and methods of the discipline are not as fixed and tidy and indisputably certain as they appear on the pages of slick textbooks. Taking students behind the scenes of the textbooks into the messy world of knowledge production and verification is the catalyst for the reflective skepticism that McPeck identifies as critical thinking.[13] However, the issue of whether thinking skills are domain specific or whether general skills can be transferred among disciplines has not been resolved. Some evidence suggests that some general thinking skills can be learned, which are applicable in several disciplines, or at least that learning such general skills makes the learning of critical thinking in a specific discipline easier.[14]

The Scientific Method

For some, critical thinking overlaps with the scientific method. Among the scientists who regard the development of thinking skills as a responsibility of science teachers are Arnold Arons and Philip J. Regal.[15] Arons, a physicist at the University of Washington and a member of the Delphi Team, suggests that to teach science the instructor must present content but also must focus on the thinking skills that are part of analysis and inquiry: raising questions and searching for evidence for answers, recognizing when answers are formulated through incomplete information or necessary leaps of faith, distinguishing inference and observation, uncovering assumptions, drawing inferences, hypothesizing conclusions, testing one's own reasoning processes. Regal, a professor of ecology and behavioral biology, in his worthwhile book *The Anatomy of Judgment* attempts to demonstrate how critically formulated judgments can serve as a bridge between science and the liberal arts. Regal's situation of critical thinking within scientific, historical, anthropological, and philosophical traditions provides a broad perspective absent in some discussions of critical thinking.

Psychology and Education

Benjamin Bloom is probably most widely referenced in critical thinking instruction and scholarship.[16] Bloom lists six levels of cognitive abilities that he believes build upon one another:

1.0 Knowledge	Recalling specific facts or general concepts	
2.0 Comprehension	Demonstrating the lowest level of understanding. The individual can make use of what is being communicated without necessarily relating it to other material or seeing its fullest implication.	
3.0 Application	Using abstractions in concrete situations. The abstractions may be principles, ideas, and theories that must be remembered and applied.	
4.0 *Analysis*	Breaking down a communication into its constituent elements. The relationships between ideas are made explicit, and the organization of the communication is understood.	
5.0 *Synthesis*	Putting together elements to form a whole—arranging elements to constitute a structure not clearly there before.	
6.0 *Evaluation*	Making judgments about the value of materials and methods for given purposes. The individual can make appraisals that satisfy criteria determined by the instructor or by others.	

Reprinted with permission of the McGraw Hill Companies. Bloom BS, Hastings JT, and Madaus GF. Handbook on formative and summative valuation of student learning. New York: McGraw-Hill, 1971:271-3.

> **Delphi Consensus on Critical Thinking Cognitive Skills and Subskills**
> *Peter Facione*
>
> 1. Interpretation
>   categorization
>   decoding significance
>   clarifying meaning
>
> 2. Analysis
>   examining ideas
>   identifying arguments
>   analyzing arguments
>
> 3. Evaluation
>   assessing claims
>   assessing arguments
>
> 4. Inference
>   querying evidence
>   conjecturing alternatives
>   drawing conclusions
>
> 5. Explanation
>   stating results
>   justifying procedures
>   presenting arguments
>
> 6. Self-regulation
>   self-examination
>   self-correction

Facione PA. Critical thinking: a statement of expert consensus for purposes of educational assessment and instruction. Washington DC: U.S. Department of Education, Office of Education Research and Improvement, 1990. (Public domain)

The last three levels, analysis, synthesis, and particularly evaluation, are often regarded as critical thinking skills. Bloom's work has been seminal, although scholars from a number of competing fields have pointed out insufficiencies in his taxonomy.

For instance, Barbara Z. Presseisen would like to see thinking models that are more descriptive and developmental.[17] She identifies four cognitive processes, categorizing critical thinking as one of four higher-order cognitive process:

Essential cognitive processes: the basic thinking skills that are the building blocks of thought development [recall, recognition, comparison, classification, inference, analogy, inductive/deductive reasoning, interpretation, evaluation]

Higher-order cognitive processes: the more complex thinking skills ... which are based on the essential cognitive processes [these involve complex reasoning, nuanced judgment, problems with non-algorithmic and multiple solutions]. The higher order processes are:

1. Problem-solving
2. Decision-making
3. Critical thinking
4. Creative thinking

Metacognitive processes: the learning to learn skills aimed at making thinking more conscious and the student more aware of the ways one can go about problem solving or decision making; [involves motivation and curiosity; knowledge of what to do when one does not comprehend]

Epistemic processes: the kind of knowledge related to particular bodies of knowledge or subject matter and the particular problems addressed by these knowledge areas ... [what is important in discipline; how does one learn and transfer and internalize; what must the student do.]

Philosophical and psychological approaches to critical thinking sometimes overlap, but there are also some fundamental differences and at times even contentiousness.[18] Psychology's approach to critical thinking naturally has tended to be more empirical and less prescriptive. More attention is given to what is happening internally in the student and to what the context of learning is. From this perspective, effective critical thinking instruction must address such questions as, what previous learning has taken place, what concepts and cognitive structures students have already formed, what misconceptions the students bring to the subject matter, how an expert solves problems differently than a novice, at what stage of development students begin to synthesize or evaluate. A basic premise is that you must know how students think before you can hope to improve their thinking.

A starting point for many researchers has been Jean Piaget's well-known classification of cognitive development into four stages: sensory-motor, preoperational, concrete operational, and formal. Each stage of development marks a qualitatively different way of thinking. The goal of critical thinking education would be to foster formal thinking, at which stage students develop the abilities to abstract, analyze, hypothesize, synthesize, and use propositional logic. Larry Little from DeKalb College, for instance, administers the Group Assessment of Logical Thinking (GALT) test to determine whether students are in a concrete, transitional, or formal stage of cognitive development so that he can devise appropriate teaching strategies for students in the earlier stages, including an emphasis on hands-on activities and on concept invention. One of the more ambitious applications of Piagetian principles is Robert Karplus' program of learning cycles, which guide students from concrete to abstract reasoning thought through phases of exploration, invention (concept formation), and application. The University of Nebraska developed this approach into a yearlong freshman program called Accent on Developing Abstract Processes of Thought (ADAPT). Researchers report significant increases in critical thinking for students who have completed the ADAPT program.[19]

Procedural Learning

Following Piaget, some theorists, particularly cognitive scientists, make a useful distinction between declarative (or figurative) learning from procedural (or operative) learning.[20] Declarative knowledge, "knowing that," refers to mastery of content, to the accumulation of facts and principles. Procedural knowledge, "knowing how," refers to the abilities to analyze the facts and principles, understand where they come from, how to apply them, and how to use them in new situations. Procedural knowledge thus encompasses critical thinking as well as creative thinking and problem-solving. Thomas A. Angelo and K. Patricia Cross' *Classroom Assessment Techniques* provides helpful concrete strategies for assessing both declarative and procedural learning.

Models of Intellectual Development

Developmental models of intellectual growth posit that a student's epistemological assumptions about such concepts as truth, authority, and objectivity are important factors in intellectual development.[21] They caution that critical thinking instruction must recognize and address these assumptions to better enable instructors to help students in their intellectual growth.

William Perry proposes that growth in critical thinking requires a person's progressive reconceptualization of what constitutes knowledge.[22] Perry interviewed male college students at Harvard to determine if their ideas of knowledge changed during the college years. To simplify Perry's model, college students appear to pass through stages of intellectual development. In the first stage, "Dualism," students tend to view the world in terms of right and wrong, black and white, and have little tolerance for ambiguity. Professors are the experts who know what reality is; the job of the student is to listen to the authority, write down what is said, and repeat it on a test. After a while students recognize that professors in different disciplines, and even within the same discipline, do not always agree. The knowledge enterprise is perceived as a tricky game with no right or wrong answers. In this second stage, "Multiplicity," students are unwilling to make normative judgments, for opinions are all that exist. In the third stage, "Relativism," students recognize that some answers are better than others if everyone agrees on criteria. Standards and procedures are keys to knowledge. If students arrive at the fourth stage of "Commitment" (apparently most do not), they recognize the need to construct and take responsibility for a world view to which they are committed but which they are willing to modify as new evidence presents itself. Facility with critical thinking is necessary to arrive at this fourth stage, but critical thinking itself does not guarantee that students will adopt such a position.

Perry's work has become the springboard for a number of studies, including one by Mary Belenky et al., who interviewed 135 women to determine if Perry's model (based upon interviews with male students) applied to the experience of women.[23] They concluded that female students pass through different stages. In fact, for many women their ways of knowing come into direct conflict with traditional methods of teaching. Women progress through stages of "Silence," or allegiance to authorities; "Received knowledge," or knowledge exists outside of self; "Subjective knowledge," or realization that they too are authorities; "Procedural knowledge," or entrance into a community forum where rational and objective standards exist; and "Constructed knowledge," or confidence and passion about one's ability to make sense of the world.

Craig Nelson, a professor of Biology at Indiana University, has adapted the work of Perry, Belenky et al., and others to develop a teaching practice that encourages students to progress in their level of critical thinking or intellectual development. Nelson's strategy is to determine the student's stage of development and then employ teaching methods that encourage and support students to make transitions to the next stage.[24] For instance, for students in the dualistic or "Sergeant Friday" stage who want "the facts, just the facts, Ma'am," he cites turning points in science, such as Newton and Euclid, when the indisputably certain turns out to be false and new scientific paradigms arise. For students in the Baskin-Robbins 31-Flavors stage in which any selection of a theory or belief is entirely subjective, like picking out a flavor of ice cream (i.e., multiplicity), he stresses precise thinking and the development of criteria for theories (consistency, data, predicatory power, etc.). As the instructor tries to nudge the student to make transitions to higher stages, he or she has an obligation to provide not only intellectual but also emotional support.

A Sample of Critical Thinking Decisions

> Critical thinking is defined in many ways. It is important to identify what you intend to emphasize when you teach critical thinking.

- Critical thinking is the intellectually disciplined process of actively and skillfully conceptualizing, applying, analyzing, synthesizing, and/or evaluating information gathered from, or generated by, observation, experience, reflection, reasoning, or communication, as a guide to belief and action. — *National Council for Excellence in Critical Thinking Instruction*

- The ability to present well-reasoned arguments and to evaluate the arguments of others. — *Peter Facione*

- Thinking is an active, purposeful, organized process which we use to make sense of the world, solve problems, work toward goals, analyze issues. Critical thinking is making sense of our world by carefully examining the thinking process in order to clarify and improve our understanding. — *John Chaffee*

- Critical consciousness of the thinking process itself and its products, a commitment to approach life in this way. — *Arts and Humanities at Alverno*

- Critical thinking is reasonable, reflective thinking that is focused on deciding what to believe or do. — *Robert Ennis*

- Knowledge, comprehension, application, analysis, synthesis, and evaluation. — *Benjamin Bloom*

- Process of inquiry involving knowledge, skills, beliefs, attitudes, and conditions directed toward forming an understanding. The outcome is an argument, interpretation, etc. — *Joanne Kurfiss*

- Purposeful, self-regulatory judgment which results in interpretation, analysis, evaluation, and inference, as well as explanation of the evidential, conceptual, methodological, criteriological, or contextual considerations upon which that judgment is based — *Delphi Consensus*

- Ability to handle abstract ideas, ambiguity, concepts, and complexity, and to make judgments; dynamic interactive stages of seeking, understanding, processing, and communicating. — *Elizabeth Hawthorne*

- The ability to actively recognize, analyze, and evaluate one's own assumptions and those of others instead of passively accepting them. — *Northeast Missouri State University*

- Asking "How do we know?" being aware of gaps in knowledge, discriminating between observation and inference, discerning the difference between ideas and their representation, probing for assumptions, drawing inferences, deductive logic, inductive logic, self-evaluating, self-consciousness of thinking. — *Arnold Arons*

Critical Thinking as an Integration of Abilities: Ability-Based Education

At Alverno College where ability-based outcomes guide the curriculum, thinking is taught and assessed not as a set of discrete skills but as an ability, i.e., an integration of knowledge, skills, and attitudes.[25] After years of study, Alverno College concluded that two basic abilities needed as a foundation for critical thinking are: **analysis** ("the process of separating and examining to distinguish constituent elements") and **communication** ("a synthesizing process" that is a way of thinking and learning).

Alverno developed a highly integrative approach to analysis and communication that involves explicit outcomes and active learning strategies. Alverno College's approach to critical thinking involves the following steps:

First, analysis and communication are broken down into a sequence of six levels. For instance, in the first two years of the curriculum, analysis means 1) observing accurately, 2) making justifiable inferences, 3) relating parts or elements in patterns, and 4) integrating patterns into coherent systems. Then in the student's major area in the last two years, analysis outcomes are 5) comparing and testing frameworks in one's discipline, and 6) integrating frameworks into a professional synthesis.

Second, for each level, criteria are established. For instance, two criteria for analysis at level 4 are: "Out of an explicit framework, articulates and distinguishes between observations, inferences, and relationships in work under investigation," and "Shows awareness of assumptions, implications, and limitations of any framework used." In every course, explicit assignments are given so that students can identify and practice the desired performance criteria.

At Alverno College, communication and analysis are components of critical thinking. Each is broken down into a sequence of six levels:

ANALYSIS	COMMUNICATION
(Levels 1–4 are covered in General Education Courses)	
1. Observes accurately	1. Assesses own communication
2. Makes justifiable inferences	2. Communicates with analytic consciousness of the process
3. Relates parts or elements in patterns	3. Communicates with effective control of the process
4. Integrates patterns into coherent systems	4. Integrates effective communication within the framework of academic disciplines
(Levels 5–6 are developed in the major)	
5. Compares and tests frameworks in one's discipline	5. Develops and applies theoretical perspectives
6. Integrates frameworks into a professional synthesis	6. Integrates communication modes effectively in professional contexts

Reprinted with permission of Alverno College©, Milwaukee, WI.

Working from the concept of assessment as learning, Alverno College provides a series of self, peer, and expert assessments to give feedback so that students can improve their performances.

Problem-Solving and Decision-Making

The terms "critical thinking" and "problem solving" are sometimes used interchangeably; sometimes they are seen as parallel activities, and sometimes one is made a subdivision of the other. The nature of the "problem" and the approach to a solution can be used as criteria to determine the relationship between the two processes. Solving problems of an algorithmic or procedural nature may involve extremely complex thinking but it need not involve critical thinking. Using astronomical observations and astrological charts to determine a marriage partner could require complicated problem-solving skills that challenge the capabilities of even a perfectly designed computer chip, but unless an evaluation of the assumptions behind the task are considered, it is unlikely that the thinking involved could be called "critical." On the other hand, critical thinking can occur in isolation from any particular problem at hand, unless the concept of "problem" is generalized to such an extent that it means any topic of intellectual interest. Even then, the critical thinker may be more interested in raising questions than in providing answers. Critical thinkers often create more problems than they solve. That is one reason the Athenians put Socrates to death.

Another way of saying this is that "problem" is not a univocal term. Problems come in many varieties and in many degrees of complexity. One way of classifying them is to place them somewhere on a continuum between "open" and "closed." A closed-ended problem has a correct answer that is verifiable; often a well-defined process can be taught for solving the problem. Figuring out why my car won't start may be a complex problem that requires a great deal of education and experience, but it is still mainly a closed-ended question. Answers to open-ended problems, like what to do about the federal deficit (or how to create a successful program in critical thinking instruction), cannot be proven to be true, and probably more than one answer could be found to solve the problem. Sometimes open-ended problems have no solution.

Kurfiss distinguishes problem solving and critical thinking by the goals they attempt: the goal of problem solving is to "find and execute a solution"; the goal of critical thinking is to "construct a plausible representation of the situation or issue that could be presented in a convincing argument."[26] Thus, critical thinking is more prevalent in the humanities and social sciences because in those disciplines arguments tend to be probabilistic rather than demonstrable. Sciences and math tend more to problem solving, especially problem solving on a hypothetico-deductive model.

But Eta S. Berner warns against unexamined assumptions that underlie paradigms of problem solving in medical education, e.g., that medical problems are relatively homogenous and generally can be solved by the hypothetico-deductive approach of science.[27] She calls for a paradigm change that allows for the identification of multiple types of problems and a corresponding set of solution processes. What is implied here is that problem solving should not be taught as one automated process; critical thinking often is necessary to determine whether a problem exists, to define the nature of the problem, and to choose an appropriate problem-solving strategy. For instance, identifying and testing assumptions is a critical thinking skill. Without such analysis of assumptions we can be controlled by paradigmatic modes of thought of which we are unaware. When faced with a medical problem, two physicians will select different strategies and arrive at different solutions if one unreflectively assumes that she needs to address the *patient's* problem and the other assumes, without recognizing an alternative, that he needs to solve the *physician's* (i.e., his own) problem. Thus problem-solving may be employed independently of critical thinking, and probably vice versa, but critical thinking nonetheless can be a powerful tool for solving problems, particularly open-ended problems.

Problem-based Learning

Problem-based learning (PBL) is an instructional approach organized around real life problems as the context for learning. It employs case studies and other traditional problem-solving activities, but it is different in that no lecturing, or a minimum amount, is used. PBL is "not simply the addition of problem-solving activities to otherwise discipline-centered curricula, but a way of conceiving of the curriculum which is centered around key problems in professional practice. Problem-based courses start with problems rather than disciplinary knowledge."[28] After being presented with a problem, such as a case study or term paper, students work in groups to analyze the problem and to determine and organize what relevant knowledge they have already. They then identify learning issues—those facts and ideas they will need to learn to solve the problem. Together, the students create a plan for learning, determine what resources will be needed, and assign responsibilities. As they meet to discuss their progress, they identify additional learning issues and revise their learning plans. PBL thus is learner-centered, individualized instruction. Faculty still have important roles in the educational process, but more as guides and resources for students rather than as information providers. Assessment is more often conducted by performance testing rather than by traditional examinations.

Three influential proponents of problem-solving educational strategies are Donald Woods from McMaster University, Charles Wales from West Virginia University, and Howard S. Barrows who did pioneering work at McMaster.

Woods counts 60 or more different problem solving strategies in the literature but finds most have the same basic steps that make up the MacMaster Problem-Solving Six Stage Strategy: read, analyze, represent internally, plan, do, look back.[29] To solve problems effectively, students must have knowledge about the subject, be able to identify and locate information that is missing, engage in self-learning, display tolerance for ambiguity, exhibit interpersonal and communication skills, develop metacognition, and value the habit of perseverance. Wales originated Guided Design, a problem-solving teaching strategy that combines case studies with a type of programmed instruction that uses printed directions to model for students a problem-solving process. The goal is for students to develop both subject matter and skills by following an 11-step process for creating solutions to open-ended problems that have more than one possible solution. The decision-making model Wales proposes has four operations: state the goal, generate ideas, prepare a plan, take action. Within each operation are the three steps of identifying problems (analysis), creating options (synthesis), and selecting a plan (evaluation).[30]

As early as the 1950s and 1960s, PBL had been adapted to medical education at Case Western Reserve University and McMaster University. It has been employed within individual courses and as a philosophy for an entire medical school curriculum, such as at Harvard and New Mexico.

Working with the McMaster System of PBL for medical education, Howard S. Barrows, M.D., proposes that in PBL medical education courses students: 1) acquire a knowledge base that is organized effectively for recall in a clinical setting and easily extended in further study; 2) develop scientific or analytic reasoning skills; 3) develop self-directed learning skills; 4) think independently and critically; 5) be sensitive to all patient needs; 6) integrate their learning; and 7) become excited about learning and motivated to undertake individualized learning. Anticipating faculty objections to a problem-solving approach, Barrows argues that PBL does not rule out also using traditional methods of teaching. Students' learning is not limited to what is directly relevant to the problem under investigation, assessment can be objective and rigorous, and the learning is time efficient. Students learn content as well as processes, and faculty do have a very important role in the learning process.[31]

After a review of PBL in medical education programs from 1972-1992, however, Mark A. Albanese and Susan Mitchell advise caution regarding implementation of problem-based learning.[32] The authors found that students in PBL generally receive a more nurturing experience that is enjoyable for both faculty and students. Compared with traditional students, PBL students do as well or better on clinical exams and faculty evaluations. However, some PBL students scored lower on basic science exams, causing concern that they may have gaps in cognitive knowledge base and a tendency toward backward reasoning. Though they acknowledge weaknesses in study design, the authors suggest that until further study can be undertaken, medical schools should consider combining instructor-directed study in the basic sciences with a PBL approach that becomes more sophisticated as the students' knowledge base increases.[33]

PBL has proven to be fertile ground for implementation in pharmacy education, being adopted in significant ways by institutions such as the University of Mississippi and the McWhorter School of Pharmacy at Samford University. While citing potential problems (such as cost, providing students with a sufficient knowledge base, and orienting students to a new method of learning) and acknowledging that additional evaluation of the method must be conducted, innovators are optimistic regarding the potential of PBL and are attempting to promote thinking development and problem-solving abilities through a student-directed learning approach.[34]

Summary

Critical thinking thus has been interrelated with analysis of arguments, problem solving, decision making, cognitive development, creativity, higher order thinking skills, the scientific method, and construction of a world view.

Though it may be easy for the classroom teacher to become disheartened or overwhelmed by the several and conflicting opinions about critical thinking, the continuing debate over what constitutes critical thinking is productive. The resulting insights and refinements should lead to better educational programs. At their best the arguments in the debate over definition can be seen as self-referential examples of what critical thinking is and also leave us with a healthy skepticism about there being only one right model or one right way to teach critical thinking within professional contexts.

Developing a program for critical thinking instruction thus demands the faculty member's informed decision-making. An uninformed decision would be to try to teach critical thinking as an activity in the last 20 minutes of class on Fridays. It needs to be integrated from the beginning stages of course planning, not tacked on as an extra. There should be a congruence among our goals, epistemological assumptions, theories of learning, curricular structures, and pedagogical methods.

If the goal is to develop lifelong abilities of inquiry and judgment, a reliance on didactic instruction as the only educational strategy is a mistake. If we believe that students' minds are not inert containers for knowledge, that instead their minds actively construct knowledge out of prior experience and through previously developed mental structures, it is a mistake to rely solely on passive learning techniques or to teach only a subject matter and not a student. If we want students to analyze and make decisions, then our teaching strategies and testing must move beyond declarative knowledge. If we want students to solve problems of increasing complexity, then we need to design curricula that are centered around the learning and practicing and improving of those skills.

Questions for Reflection

Here is a list of questions you can use to analyze your goals and strategies so as to integrate critical thinking into didactic and experiential learning experiences.

1. Is it sufficient in my course/experiential learning for students to learn content, or are they expected to be able to do something with the content? What must they do? What thinking skills are required for them to do it?
2. What discrete thinking skills are most important for my course?
3. Are students required in my course to analyze? to synthesize? to evaluate? Should they be? Where specifically in the course are they required to perform these activities? What could be done?
4. Is it important in my class/clinical site for students to learn how to solve problems within my discipline? What problems are there to solve? What instruction are they given to do so? In what ways do they practice solving problems? What feedback do I give them?
5. Do I have a responsibility to help students develop a deeper understanding of their thinking, to expand their understanding of knowledge, or to broaden and deepen their world views?
6. What are the conventions of my discipline; what counts as evidence or what makes for convincing arguments? Is it important in my teaching for students to recognize the conventions of my discipline, to determine what counts as evidence or what makes for convincing arguments? If yes, how do I teach these things?
7. Is it important for me to adopt my teaching strategies to various learning styles and to various levels of intellectual development?
8. Do I have a responsibility to try to motivate students to value knowledge, to be inquisitive, to seek truth, to tolerate ambiguity?
9. In what ways do I model critical thinking for my students? In what ways could I?
10. What types of support do I give my students as they are developing critical thinking skills and attitudes? What types of support should I be giving?

11. What percentage of my test questions require memory? What percentage require comprehension? What percentage require higher order critical thinking skills? Are these percentages appropriate for my course goals?
12. What definition(s) and model(s) of higher order thinking skills can best facilitate my preparation and teaching of critical thinking?
13. What one change in my teaching would be most effective in helping students develop better thinking skills? What would it take to implement it?

Notes

1. Integrity in the college curriculum: a report to the academic community. Project on Redefining the Meaning and Purpose of Baccalaureate Degrees. Washington DC : Association of American Colleges, 1985.
2. Bootman JL, Garnett WR, Miller WA, Ryan MR, Spratto GR. Components of a minimum college curriculum: relationship to pharmacy education. White paper from the 1985-86 Academic Affairs Committee. Am J Pharm Educ 1986;50:386-9.
3. Chalmers RK, Gibson RD, Schumacher GE, Sorby DL, Zografi G. Liberal education—a key structural component in pharmacy education. Report of the 1986-1987 Argus Commission. Am J Pharm Educ 1987;51:446-50.
4. Cohen JL, Chair Report for the Academic Affairs Committee. Am J Pharm Educ 1988; 52:409-11.
5. American Association of Colleges of Pharmacy. Background Paper II: Entry-Level, Curricular Outcomes, Curricular Content and Educational Process [1990]. Commission to Implement Change in Pharmaceutical Education. Am J Pharm Educ 1993;57:17, 20.
6. For instance, see Miller DR. An assessment of critical thinking: can pharmacy students evaluate clinical studies like experts? Am J Pharm Educ 2004;68(1):article 5. Miller DR. Longitudinal assessment of critical thinking in pharmacy students. Am J Pharm Educ 2003;67:article 120. Monaghan MS, Vanderbush RE, McKay AB, Gardner SF, Schneider EF. A computerized database approach to enhance critical thinking. J Pharm Teach 1999;7:35-50. Phillips CR, Chesnut RJ, Rospond RM. The California critical thinking instruments for benchmarking, program assessment, and directing curricular change. Am J Pharm Educ 2004;68: article 101. Austin Z, Boyd C. Development of a sequenced strategic thinking assignment syllabus for a senior-level professional practice course. Am J Pharm Educ 1998;62:119-23. Adamcik B, Hurley S, Erramouspe J. Assessment of pharmacy students' critical thinking and problem-solving abilities. Am J Pharm Educ 1996;60:256-65. Zlatic TD, Nowak DM, Sylvester D. Integrating general and professional education through a study of herbal products: an intercollegiate collaboration. Am J Pharm Educ 2000;64:83-94. Hobson EH, Schafermeyer KW. Writing and critical thinking: writing-to-learn in large classes. Am J Pharm Educ 1994;58:423-27. Haworth IS, Eriksen SP, Chmait SH, et al. Use of computer-based case studies in a problem-solving curriculum. Am J Pharm Educ 1997;61:97-102. Harris FK, Harrold MW, Giudici RA, et al. Development and implementation of critical thinking assignments throughout a pharmacy curriculum. Am J Pharm Educ 1997;61:1-11. Hartzema AG. Teaching therapeutic reasoning through the case-study approach: adding the probabilistic dimension. Am J Pharm Educ 1994;58:436-40. Hunter KA. Poster presentations: an alternative to the traditional classroom lecture. Am J Pharm Educ 1997;61:78-80. Robertson KE, McDaniel AM. Interdisciplinary professional education: a collaborative clinical teaching project. Am J Pharm Educ 1995;59:131-6.
7. Allen DD, Bond CA. Prepharmacy predictors of success in pharmacy school: grade point averages, pharmacy college admissions test, communication abilities, and critical thinking skills. Pharmacotherapy 2001;21(7):842-9.

8. Paul R. Critical thinking: what every person needs to survive in a rapidly changing world. Rohnert Park, CA: Center for Critical Thinking and Moral Critique, 1990.
9. Facione PA. Critical thinking: a statement of expert consensus for purposes of educational assessment and instruction. Washington DC: U.S. Department of Education, Office of Education Research and Improvement, 1990.
10. Ennis RH. A concept of critical thinking. Harv Educ Review 1962;32:81-111.
11. McPeck J. Critical thinking and education. New York: St. Martin's Press, 1981.
12. McPeck JE. Stalking beasts, but swatting flies: the teaching of critical thinking. Can J Educ 1984;93:28-44.
13. Paul, p. 411.
14. Kurfiss JG. Critical thinking: theory, research, practice, and possibilities. ASHE-ERIC Higher Education Report No. 2. College Station, TX: Association for the Study of Higher Education, 1988.
15. Arons AB. A guide to introductory physics teaching. New York: John Wiley and Sons, 1990; and Regal PJ. The anatomy of judgment. Minneapolis: University of Minnesota Press, 1990.
16. Bloom BS, Hastings JT, Madaus GF. Handbook on formative and summative valuation of student learning. New York: McGraw-Hill, 1971:271-3.
17. Presseisen BZ. Thinking skills: research and practice. Washington DC: National Education Association, 1986.
18. Paul, p. 450.
19. Examples and background are provided in Karplus R. Science teaching and the development of reasoning. Berkeley, CA: University of California, 1977. See also Meyers C. Teaching students to think critically. San Francisco: Jossey-Bass 1986:26-39. Stonewater JK. Strategies for problem solving. In: Young RE, ed. Fostering critical thinking. San Francisco: Jossey-Bass, 1980:33-43.
20. Arons, p. 314; Anderson JR. Cognitive psychology and its implications. San Francisco: W.H. Freeman and Co., 1980. Lawson AE. The reality of general cognitive operations. Sc Educ 1982;66:229-41. Angelo TA, Cross PK. Classroom assessment techniques. San Francisco: Jossey-Bass, 1993:119.
21. Kurfiss, p. 51.
22. Perry WG Jr. Forms of intellectual and ethical development in the college years: a scheme. New York: Holt, Rinehart and Winston, 1970.
23. Belenky M, Clinchy B, Goldberger N, Tarule J. Women's ways of knowing. New York: Basic Books, 1986:101-30.
24. Nelson CE. Skewered on the unicorn's horn: the illusion of tragic tradeoff between content and critical thinking in the teaching of science. In Crow LW, ed. Enhancing critical thinking in the sciences. Washington DC: Society for College Science Teachers, 1989.
25. Loacker G, Cromwell L, Fey J, Rutherford D. Analysis and Communication at Alverno: an approach to critical thinking. Milwaukee: Alverno Productions, 1984:1. Georgine Loacker from Alverno College served as consultant to the AACP Focus Group on Liberalization of the Professional Curriculum, Chaired by Robert Chalmers. Ability-based education is explored in more detail in Chapter 6.
26. Kurfiss, p. 28.
27. Berner ES. Paradigms and problem-solving: a literature review. J Med Educ 1984:59(8):625-33.
28. Boud D, Feletti G, eds. The challenge of problem based learning. New York: St. Martin's Press, 1991:14. For an overview in pharmacy, see Jang R, Solad SW. Teaching pharmacy students problem-solving: theory and present status. Am J Pharm Educ 1990:54;161-66.

29. Woods DR. The MPS strategy book. Hamilton, Canada: McMaster University, 1992.
30. Wales CE, Stager RA, Long TR. Guided engineering design. St. Paul, MN: West, 1974. Wales CE, Nardi AH, Stager RH. Professional decision making. Morgantown, WV: Center for Guided Design, West Virginia University, 1986. Wales CE, Nardi AH, Stager RA. Decision making: new paradigm for education. Educ Leadership 1986;43:37-41.
31. Barrows HS. How to design a problem-based curriculum for the preclinical years. New York: Springer, 1985:53-4;104-12. The McMaster approach is also described in Rangachari PK. Design of a problem-based undergraduate course in pharmacology: implications for the teaching of physiology. Am J Physiol 1991;260:S14-S21.
32. Albanese MA, Mitchell S. Problem-based learning: a review of literature on its outcomes and implementation issues. Acad Med 1993;68:52-81.
33. See also Des Marchais JE, Dumais B. Issues in implementing a problem-based learning curriculum at the University of Sherbrooke. Ann of Community-oriented Educ 1990;3:9-23. Whitman N, Schwenk TS. Problem solving in medical education: can it be taught? Curr Surg 1986;43:453-9. Van Berkel HJM. Assessment in a problem-based medical curriculum. Higher Education 1990(2);19:123-46. For a general overview, see Woods DR. In Gabel D ed. Problem solving: what research says to the teacher. Vol. 5. Washington DC: National Teachers Association, 1989:97-121.
34. Eck JC. Assessing and researching problem-based learning. Birmingham, AL: Samford University Press, 2002. Monk-Tutor MR. Overview of MSOP curriculum and adoption of PBL. PBL Insight. 2003;6(1). For an overview of PBL in pharmacy see Cisneros RM, Salisbury-Glennon JD, Anderson-Harper HM. Status of problem-based learning research in pharmacy education: a call for future research. Am J Pharm Educ 2002;66:19-26. See the examples cited in Chapter 5 below; also see Fisher RC. The potential for a problem-based learning. Am J Pharm Educ 1994;58:183-9. Kaufman DM, Mann KV. Students' perceptions about their courses in problem-based-learning and conventional curricula. Acad Med. 1996:71:s52-s54.

Chapter 4: Teaching Critical Thinking within Professional Contexts

Critical thinking involves more than skills, more than techniques, more than problem solving. Critical thinking is not just a subject, a tool, or a strategy. It is an orientation. To incorporate critical thinking into pharmacy education involves broadening professional education beyond a traditional concept of classroom and clinical experience.

Critical thinking, in part, is what distinguishes education from training. Training should not be undervalued. Knowing the names of things, following procedures, recognizing problems, providing solutions, espousing professional values: these are essential skills that a professional must be trained to perform correctly. Education requires learners not only to receive and practice knowledge, but also to question, test, and modify it. These learners want to know not only the procedure but also the reasons behind it and the possibilities for improving it. They have the skills, values, and attitudes that give them the confidence to look behind conventional wisdom and to create alternative ideas and strategies. Critical thinking is a term that represents the integration of this knowledge, skills, attitudes, and values.

Critical thinking education fits in with the "learning as growth" paradigm that views learning as transformative rather than simply accretive. Learning produces qualitative as well as quantitative changes.[1] Critical thinking in this model is metacognitive; i.e., it involves an awareness, critique, and correction of our thinking processes. It involves a predisposition to seek evidence and arguments before assenting to any propositions or beliefs. Enemies of critical thinking are ignorance, naïveté, complacency, pomposity, manipulation, uncritical acceptance of tradition. The tasks of the critical thinker are to find and understand information; to analyze it and the assumptions upon which it is based; to determine its accuracy, fairness, and relevance; to recognize the reliability of observations and the cogency of arguments; to identify and establish criteria to evaluate ideas; to make sound judgments; to arrive at correct conclusions; to create new alternatives and ideas.

Critical Thinking: Knowledge, Skills, and Attitudes, Habits, Values

Sometimes it is assumed that there is a tension between teaching content and teaching abilities such as critical thinking. Pharmacy education involves learning huge chunks of basic content from multiple disciplines in the chemical, biological, pharmaceutical, and administrative sciences. Many of these courses are introductory in nature. The amount of material needed to be taught puts pressure on instructors to convey information quickly and efficiently. Although the evolution of professional practice requires students to acquire increasing facility with procedural knowledge, they still need to possess massive amounts of declarative knowledge. Taking time to analyze or evaluate information, some instructors fear, may mean that some information will not be taught in the classroom. Also, the introductory level of many courses means that in some disciplines students do not have an extensive knowledge base from which to make informed judgments or even to ask probing questions.

But this is a false dilemma. If you were going to have brain surgery, would you choose a surgeon who is so skilled with a scalpel she can slice a fly's eye into 18 equal parts but who can't always remember where the neocortex is, or the surgeon who can cite every article on Medline but who drops his fork on the floor three times during lunch? Even in these days of managed health care, most of us would look for a third alternative. Knowledge is a prerequisite for critical thinking. Without knowledge, one cannot uncover hidden assumptions, recognize errors, analyze arguments, or solve problems. To ignore content in order to teach thinking would be shallow and self-defeating. And vice versa, for teaching content apart from thinking tends to lead not to knowledge but to transmission of information that may not be remembered for very long.

Some efficiency-minded instructors pressured by a need to transmit huge databases of facts to students would prefer that students be rounded up into one course where they would be taught critical thinking once and for all so that when they get to the real pharmacy courses no one would have to mess with it. There is evidence to suggest this one-time effort won't work.[2] Perhaps some generalized critical thinking skills can be applied across disciplines, but to some extent at least, the critical thinking process seems to be dependent upon disciplinary knowledge. Put five Ph.D. philosophers into a antimicrobial pharmacotherapy course and see what kind of response they can give when asked to use their critical thinking skills to recommend or evaluate a therapy. Although their response may be more logical than another group equally ignorant of disease states and medications, without knowledge of the facts, ideas, rules, assumptions, values, and methodologies of the discipline, it is unlikely they would be considered effective critical thinkers in that area.

Thus critical thinking instruction does not devalue content but makes the learning of content even more urgent. The required content now involves not only discrete facts but also knowledge of the disciplinary rules and conventions so that students can process the facts effectively. The goal is to give students not just the facts of biology or chemistry or pharmacy, but also the knowledge needed to think as a biologist or chemist or pharmacist.

In addition, if students are going to learn to think and reason better, they need some knowledge about thinking and reasoning within their discipline. When asked at faculty development programs, "Who teaches critical thinking in their courses or practice experiences?" almost every faculty member's hand goes up. When asked what they do in their course to teach critical thinking, some are more pressed to give answers. Critical thinking should not just be *required* in courses; it should be explicitly *taught*. A first step is to ensure that students understand terminology such as inductive and deductive thinking,

> Educational reformers posit that by supporting students in directing their own learning and providing them the tools they need to access, analyze, and apply information, education will be transformed.
>
> *Health Professions Education: A Bridge to Quality.*
> *Institute of Medicine*

inferences, assumptions, analysis, evaluation. (It would be an interesting experiment to determine how many fourth-year college students could give an adequate definition of synthesis, much less actually synthesize.) Introducing Bloom's taxonomy or Piaget's stages or Perry's scheme of intellectual development can help students develop facts and conceptual frameworks to guide their learning.

Secondly, an attempt to develop critical thinking should focus on discrete thinking skills. Students need explicit instruction, for instance, on how to analyze (compare/contrast, classify), distinguish facts from assumptions, make and evaluate inferences, reason deductively and inductively, recognize fallacies and inconsistencies, hypothesize, interpret, evaluate, synthesize, diagnose, solve problems, and make decisions. They must be able to recognize and apply criteria to be able to evaluate when these skills are practiced successfully. Of course in professional education these skills are exercised within the context of professional abilities: Students improve their thinking skills in the process of learning to select or monitor drug therapy or assess patient disease states.

Further, teaching critical thinking involves more than a body of knowledge and a set of skills. A critical thinker also adopts critical attitudes, dispositions, and habits—the skill to think well as well as the willingness and desire to do so. Critical thinking has affective components: enhanced thinking skills will not be productive without the courage to test one's beliefs, the humility to admit to error, the passion to seek truth, the joy of discovery, a tolerance for ambiguity. And there is even an ethical component. Critical thinking is not simply a set of mechanical, cognitive skills to be employed for sophistical argument, economic gain, or self-aggrandizing games of one-upmanship. Without maturity of mind, intellectual honesty, openness, and breadth of perspective, critical thinking becomes simply another sleight-of-mind trick rather than a force for intellectual progress and personal freedom. Critical thinking education cannot ignore the affective and ethical domains.

Thus, a critical thinking program should attempt to foster habits, attitudes, and values that are conducive to higher order thinking. Excitement about learning, intellectual integrity, and unrelenting self-examination, it is true, are outcomes that cannot easily be taught or assessed. Faculty can invite discussion of such issues in the classroom, for instance, by calling attention to ethical implications of course material. As an example, in a pharmacy that provides pharmaceutical care and is responsible for patient information and drug education, is it proper to sell at the cash register tabloids whose headlines announce "wonder drugs" that can cure Alzheimers, toothaches, and baldness?

The instructor can appeal to the idealism latent in most students but too often left dormant in pharmacy education, where sometimes a most commonly heard motivation for choosing a pharmaceutical career is the starting salary. The instructor can try to capture the imagination of students by pointing out unexplored areas of knowledge and routes into

> When entering college our students are bright, motivated to learn, and wanting to do good for patient care. With time, our students become brow-beaten, cynical, and survival, not lifelong learning, is their desire. This is why we must take the opportunity to change how we educate our students, and to turn them on to the liberating excitement of learning.
>
> *Nick Popovich*

that unknown territory to be taken by adventurous minds. Students need to be rigorously challenged in their course work, not with tedious tasks but with meaningful assignments that add to their knowledge base and also invite them to reconsider how they see or think or do. Students can at least be given the tools that will enable lifelong learning, and for some that is encouragement enough.

Instructors can devise a variety of teaching strategies, course activities, and projects that are both challenging and interesting. One strategy would be to redesign assessment practices. Summative assessment is of course necessary, but too often it promotes cramming for tests with the goal of passing the course rather than understanding the material. Formative assessment encourages learning, a process for recognizing weaknesses and opportunities for correcting them (this is discussed in Chapter 6).

Modeling and mentoring are most effective in shaping student attitudes. Students respond to the instructor's excitement in the classroom, to an obvious passion for learning, to a willingness to acknowledge mistakes, and to a commitment to research, publication, and other scholarly activities that extend beyond a worry over promotion and tenure. The instructor's demonstration of professional values is more convincing than a classroom lecture on professionalism. The instructor who shows concern and support for students, who practices "educational care," is more likely to help students understand the implications of "pharmaceutical care."[3]

Critical thinking, then, is not something simply to be inserted into a curriculum; instead, it is an orientation, an organizing principle. Linda Salamon, then dean of Washington University's College of Arts and Sciences, proposed that integrity, or "wholeness," in the professional curriculum is achieved when the exercise of inquiry and judgment is pursued along with in-depth knowledge. In terms of critical inquiry and study in depth, Salamon asked pharmacy faculty to evaluate their teaching according the following criteria:

- Do your courses teach students not facts but the power to establish facts, to bring them together as evidence, to prove the apparent results, to let imagination and even intuition play over them? Do you let students draw their own conclusions, including (on occasion) false ones?

- And in your professional studies, do you strengthen those critical and analytic powers and invite students to make their own syntheses? Or just to accept yours? Do you reveal to them how little we know about drug action? How often new discoveries prove our assumptions wrong? Do they learn the humility in the limits of your profession? Do they question its economics, its marketing, its role in preventive health-care? Do you stuff them full of today's evanescent knowledge, at the expense of liberating powers of reasoning and application? 80 credits, presented (to my eye) as training rather than education, suggest that you may. I cannot be sure; I don't know what happens inside courses like industrial pharmaceutical technology or psychopharmacology, but I wonder.[4]

Pharmacy faculty in didactic courses and experiential education who want to produce graduates with healthy skepticism and critical, questioning minds should keep these questions in mind as they address issues of content, skills, and attitudes.

This is not to imply that critical thinking instruction is a novelty or innovation in pharmacy education. In fact, pharmacy educators have been leaders in higher education in

> I have this romantic idea of teaching as gift exchanges. What matters is if I reach a few students at a level that transforms them and gets them to see the world in a different way. Gift exchanges. Sure teaching is method and information, but it's something else, a gift, an enrichment of your life, a transformation that you spend the rest of your life discovering.
>
> P.F. Kluge

transforming learning so that it incorporates active learning strategies for achieving higher order thinking. Nor is it meant to imply that traditional methods of education must be scrapped. Lectures are an effective, economical method of conveying large amounts of information to many people in a short amount of time. Memorization is indispensable for laying a groundwork of knowledge (our most basic technique for information retrieval, alphabetical order, can be known only by rote memory). Objective testing helps to assess whether students have grasped basic information. In other words, pharmacy education has a variety of goals and needs a variety of teaching strategies. If critical thinking is to be one of these goals, it must be built into the planning for the course and curriculum in order to ensure that students develop the knowledge, skills, and motivation to become independent, lifelong learners who can think critically, solve problems, and make responsible decisions. What should be clear is that critical thinking instruction involves more than a series of quick-fix techniques that can be inserted as add-ons or afterthoughts to an already packed course. It requires a rethinking of goals and practices.

Getting Started: Using Bloom to Teach Higher Levels of Thinking

A relatively simple way to begin teaching toward higher level thinking skills is to use Bloom's taxonomy as a framework when designing assignments and tests.

Bloom states that thinking skills build upon one another. At the foundational level, a student must know—i.e., be able to recall or memorize information; objective testing is a good way to measure such knowledge. Comprehension requires students to recall and also to understand, to be able to paraphrase, for instance. Application means that the student can relate the information to new contexts. The last three levels, analysis, synthesis, evaluation, are higher order thinking skills. Analysis is the ability to take things apart, to understand

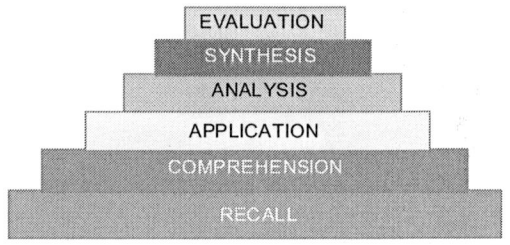

THINKING SKILLS

Benjamin Bloom

structure, to see how things fit together. Synthesis is the ability to put things together, to cull ideas from several sources, and to come up with something new. Evaluation is the determination of worth or goodness or correctness.

Working from this taxonomy, faculty can identify for themselves the expectations they have for their students regarding thinking so that they can then make conscious decisions regarding the levels of thinking they wish to assess through tests and assignments. Additionally, if students are made aware of Bloom's classification and are taught what each of the levels means, they will be able to perform better on those tests and assignments.

One way to do that is to point out to students that often the verb in the directions for an assignment or test question is a clue to what type of thinking activity is required for satisfactory performance. For instance, directions that begin with "list," "match," and "name" usually do not require students to move beyond the level of recall, whereas directions that begin with "compare" or "classify" should prompt the student that analytical skills are needed to address this assignment. To help students internalize the differences between levels of thinking skills, instructors can require an exercise in which students create sample test questions for each level of Bloom's taxonomy. Of course familiarity with the taxonomy is only a first step. An additional responsibility of the instructor is to make sure that students know how to perform these thinking tasks. The faculty member should make conscious efforts 1) to inform students what analysis, synthesis, and evaluation mean in his or her discipline; 2) to model these operations; 3) to clarify the criteria by which to judge whether or not the operations are performed well; and 4) to give examples of both successful and unsuccessful attempts.

Using Bloom, the instructor can also review previous assignments and test questions to determine what percentage of them involves recall, understanding, application, analysis, synthesis, and evaluation. Then the instructor can determine whether or not that percentage is appropriate for the course outcomes selected. If the faculty member has determined that critical thinking is a course outcome but the test questions are 80% recall, the assessments probably are not supporting the outcomes.

Asking the Right Questions

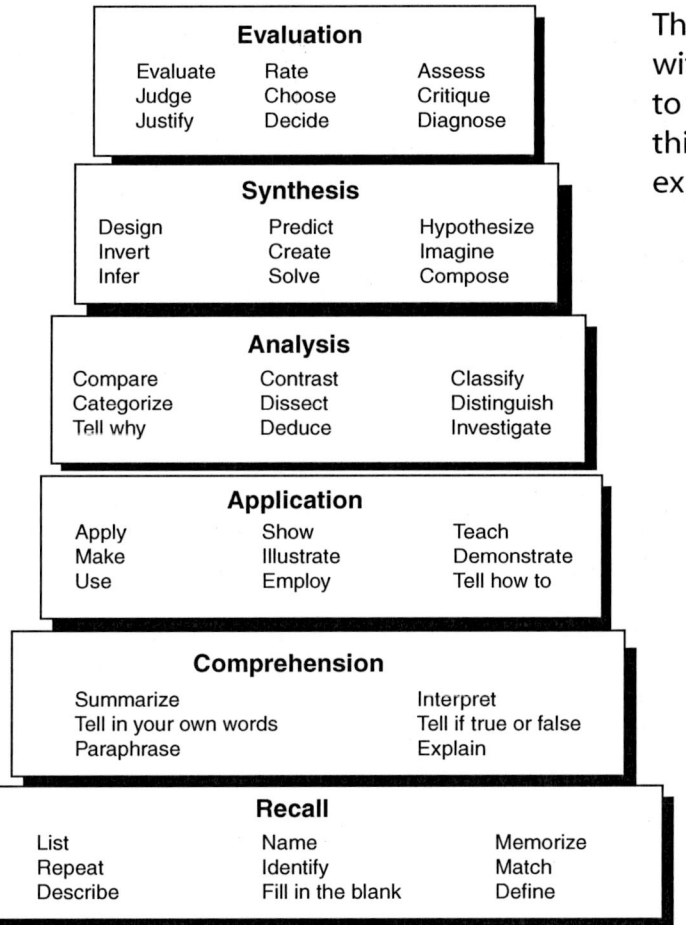

The verb you start with can be a clue to the level of thinking you are expecting.

Evaluation
- Evaluate
- Judge
- Justify
- Rate
- Choose
- Decide
- Assess
- Critique
- Diagnose

Synthesis
- Design
- Invert
- Infer
- Predict
- Create
- Solve
- Hypothesize
- Imagine
- Compose

Analysis
- Compare
- Categorize
- Tell why
- Contrast
- Dissect
- Deduce
- Classify
- Distinguish
- Investigate

Application
- Apply
- Make
- Use
- Show
- Illustrate
- Employ
- Teach
- Demonstrate
- Tell how to

Comprehension
- Summarize
- Tell in your own words
- Paraphrase
- Interpret
- Tell if true or false
- Explain

Recall
- List
- Repeat
- Describe
- Name
- Identify
- Fill in the blank
- Memorize
- Match
- Define

Using Bloom's Taxonomy to Ask Questions[5]

1. Topic: Pneumonia

Recall

| Name |
| Identify |
| List |
| Match |

List the most likely pathogen(s) responsible for community-acquired pneumonia in a 66-year-old adult smoker.

Comprehension

| Summarize |
| Interpret |
| Explain |
| Define |

A 44-year-old patient suffering from a chronic, uncontrolled seizure disorder presents to the emergency room (ER) with a 3-day history of cough and malaise. Five days prior to his presentation to the ER the patient experienced a generalized tonic-clonic seizure with loss of consciousness. Physical exam reveals a temperature of 100.5 degrees F, normal respiratory rate and diminished bilateral breath sounds. Chest x-ray is remarkable for bilateral lower lobe infiltrates.

Interpret this clinical picture:
A. Pneumococcal pneumonia
B. Aspiration pneumonia
C. Viral pneumonia
D. All of the above
E. None of the above

Application

| Apply |
| Use |
| Solve |
| Illustrate |

Apply your knowledge of pneumonia to suggest appropriate empiric antimicrobial therapy for a 55-year-old patient who presents with a typical, lobar pneumonia.

Analysis

| Compare |
| Classify |
| Outline |
| Diagram |

A 45-year-old patient with type 1 diabetes mellitus, chronic renal failure, hypertension, and coronary artery disease is hospitalized with pneumonia. The present illness has lasted approximately 1 week and is characterized by malaise, low-grade fever, and nonproductive cough without any episodes of shaking chills. The patient is hemodialyzed three times weekly and last underwent dialysis yesterday. Vital signs reveal a BP of 160/100, fever of 100 degrees F and a normal respiratory rate. Pulmonary exam is unremarkable. The patient currently has a serum potassium of 7.0 mEq/L, serum bicarbonate of 15 mEq/L, and anion gap of 16. Chest x-ray is consistent with a bilateral interstitial pneumonia. Upon interviewing other household members, you learn that the patient's 19-year-old son has suffered from a chronic nonproductive cough and low-grade fever for the past 3 weeks.

Deduce the most likely pathogen(s) responsible for this patient's pneumonia.

Synthesis

| Design |
| Create |
| Imagine |
| Modify |

Design an appropriate empiric antimicrobial regimen for the patient described in question 4 above. Include dose(s) and duration of antibiotic treatment.

Evaluation

| Assess |
| Choose |
| Evaluate |
| Justify |

Justify your answer to question 5 above by logically outlining the reasons for each antibiotic choice and dose. Provide an alternative therapy if your first choice fails or is not tolerated by the patient.

Critical Thinking Instruction in Pharmacy

We have seen that critical thinking can entail:

- Thinking about thinking in order to improve thinking
- Analyzing and critiquing ideas and situations
- Developing well-reasoned arguments with convincing evidence
- Making clinical decisions
- Solving problems
- Developing a mature world view

The challenge to the professional educator is to create opportunities so that students can practice and master these abilities within professional contexts.

The first step is to adopt thinking as a learning outcome and to construct criteria for what it means to think critically in a particular course or experiential activity. Then teaching strategies and assessments should be adopted to support that outcome. The next chapters give some examples of active learning strategies structured to achieve various learning outcomes, but a few possibilities for critical thinking can be mentioned here.

Critical thinkers often display a habit of healthy skepticism. They do not immediately accept stated facts but instead ask questions about assumptions, relevance, logic, and evidence. Socratic questioning can be employed in lectures, discussion sessions, and preceptor mentoring to stimulate such a questioning attitude. The Socratic questioner often begins by asking a seemingly simple or direct question or by responding to a student question with another question. The purpose of the questions is to guide students through a thought process. The skilled Socratic questioner leads students in uncovering assumptions and biases that they were not aware of, envisioning consequences that they had not foreseen, recognizing complexities in what seemed basic, and finding patterns in what appeared to be chaotic. The power of the technique is that the students are not told the answers but discover them through the skillful prompts of the questioner. In the encounter they begin to appreciate and internalize the investigative thought process.

Debate is another strategy to help students understand the complexity, ambiguity, and open-endedness of their discipline. When debating appropriate treatment, selection of a drug therapy, or the issue of a pharmacist's right to withhold services based on personal moral beliefs, students learn about drugs and drug therapies but also about how to find, comprehend, analyze, synthesize, and evaluate information. One innovative approach employed by residents teaching a module on Evidence-based Cardiology Medications was to create a *Law and Order* scenario in which a plaintiff was suing a hospital for malpractice regarding drug therapy. Students assumed the roles of plaintiff, prosecutor, defense lawyer, expert witnesses, judge, and jury. Everyone in the class was involved in some way in the constructing, analyzing, and evaluating evidence. Similarly, instructors can invite to class speakers who differ in their recommendations regarding drug therapies for particular disease states or patients so that students are encouraged to evaluate evidence. Along the same lines, instructors can assign medically related articles that contradict one another. In another variation, some students are assigned an article that supports use of a drug, and other students are assigned another article that argues against the use of the drug; the two groups then must debate the topic. Journal clubs and evidence-based medicine reports can also be structured to stimulate interactions that promote critical thinking.

Early in their education students should be assigned cases that are fairly straightforward, with limited complexity and with one clear solution. Faculty can teach students how to "process" a case by initially walking them through some well-constructed sample cases and identifying key pieces of information. But as students progress through the curriculum, the instructor can challenge them with complex cases that are more ambiguous, that have multiple problems for which there are competing alternative solutions, and that raise ethical dilemmas that cannot be resolved through the application of a formula. These cases should include irrelevant data or distracting "noise" so that students understand that real patients present with a mixture of data, some that will be relevant and some that will be irrelevant to the primary problem(s). Also, examples where a single piece of case data "doesn't fit" can be presented to the students for explanation in order to teach the concept of spurious findings. For example, an isolated serum potassium of 7.5 mEq/liter in a patient without any underlying renal disease, metabolic disorder, or identifiable potassium intake can be used discuss the occurrence of inaccurate electrolyte determinations that occur when a patient's blood sample is hemolyzed. The instructor needs to be careful not to confuse or overwhelm the student. In all of these activities it is important not only to *require* critical thinking but also to *teach* it, to provide instruction and assessment feedback to help students develop strategies and willingness to uncover and test assumptions, weigh evidence, apply their professional knowledge, evaluate alternatives, and make decisions that are rational, appropriate, ethical, and justified.

In-basket activities simulate the responsibilities of a pharmacist in particular practice environments. Scenarios can be created that require students to analyze ambiguous situations and make clinical decisions. The instructor then can perform follow-up assessments that provide feedback explicitly directed at the thinking process. An Objective Structured Clinical Examination (OSCE) is a more formal simulation in which students rotate through a series of clinical stations interacting with real or standardized patients, solving clinical problems while a preceptor observes and later provides assessment feedback. Service learning and reflective journals can encourage the development of an expanded world view. And of course, the purpose of exploratory laboratories, Problem-based Learning, Guided Design, and early practice experiences is to require students to reflect and act upon their learning as they observe, formulate hypotheses, research, analyze, synthesize, evaluate, and solve problems.

To become critical thinkers, students must practice critical thinking. Critical thinking instruction requires some form of active learning.

What Questions Are You Asking?

This short exercise asks you to apply your knowledge of Bloom's levels of thinking. Check your responses against the completed worksheet that follows.
1. Choose a topic from your class or practice site. _____
2. For each level of thinking, write test questions, discussion questions, or assignments regarding your topic. Use the sample or similar verbs as prompts.

Recall

| Name
| Identify
| List
| Match

_____
_____
_____

Comprehension

| Summarize
| Interpret
| Explain
| Define

_____
_____
_____

Application

| Apply
| Use
| Solve
| Illustrate

_____
_____
_____

Analysis

| Compare
| Classify
| Outline
| Diagram

_____
_____
_____

Synthesis

| Design
| Create
| Imagine
| Predict

_____
_____
_____

Evaluation

| Assess
| Choose
| Evaluate
| Justify

_____
_____
_____

3. Use Bloom's Taxonomy to evaluate a recent exam. What percentage of questions fit into each category of the Taxonomy? Is that ratio appropriate for your goals?

Remember: It is often appropriate to use lower-level thinking questions, depending upon the purpose of the assignment and course. Not every question needs to test higher order thinking.

4. Use Bloom's Taxonomy to evaluate what level of thinking is encouraged by your classroom activities. What classroom strategies could be adopted to raise the level of thinking required for the class? (See the next chapter for a list of active learning strategies.)

Notes

1. Gregory MW. Critical thinking and liberal education. Perspectives 1988;18:19-20.
2. See McPeck J. Critical thinking and education. New York: St. Martin's Press, 1981.
3. For the idea of "educational care," see Popovich NG. The educational care of pharmacy. Am J Pharm Educ 1991;55:349-55; and Becker ES, Schafermeyer KW. Educational care 101: prerequisite for pharmaceutical care. J Pharm Teach 1993;3:3-14.
4. Salamon LB. Integrity in the pharmacy curriculum. Am J Pharm Educ 1985;49:363. See also Stark JS, Lowther MA. Exploring common ground in liberal and professional education. New directions for teaching and learning 1989;40:7-20; and Dumbleton SM and Soleau JK. Liberal studies and the pharmacy curriculum: the Importance of integration. Am J Pharm Educ 1991;55:59-64.
5. This exercise was completed by Michael Maddux.

Chapter 5: Holding a Cat by the Tail: Active Learning

A Pop Quiz!

Circle the most appropriate response(s) to each question. You have 10 minutes.

1. Which students are likely to do better on a test:
   a. Students who go to class but don't review their notes before the test
   b. Students who don't go to class but review the notes of someone who did attend

2. Which procedure is mostly likely to lead to student mastery of a subject:
   a. Teaching pharmacology
   b. Teaching Helen
   c. Teaching pharmacology to Helen

3. Which of the following are **NOT** characteristic of lectures:
   a. Ability of speaker to communicate enthusiasm
   b. Ability to present material not otherwise available
   c. Ability to organize material in a special way
   d. Ability to convey large amounts of information
   e. Ability to communicate simultaneously with many people
   f. Ability to model how to attack a problem
   g. Ability to control a class
   h. Little threat to students
   i. Student attention stays high for 50 minutes
   j. Students receive sufficient feedback
   k. Excellent way to encourage higher order thinking skills
   i. Excellent way to communicate complex abstract information

4. The best reason to use active learning is:
   a. It provides immediate feedback to students
   b. It encourages critical thinking
   c. It enhances retention of content
   d. It increases student motivation

5. The best analogy for education is:
   a. filling a bucket
   b. lighting a fire

6. T F Pausing for two minutes three times during a lecture can lead to significantly better student performance on free-recall quizzes and comprehensive tests — enough for up to two letter grades difference.

7. T F Many people retain only about 10% of what they hear and up to 90% of what they say and do.

8. T F Because the average person can hold only 5-7 bits in memory, it is important to act upon the information to save it to long term memory.

9. T F Active learning strategies are not effective in large classes.

10. T F Most students resist active learning strategies.

11. T F Active learning is more likely than lecture to motivate students and to call attention to attitudes and values.

12. T F Employment of active learning strategies results in less coverage of content.

13. T F "Collaborative learning" is a name for what used to be called cheating.

14. T F On average, students after one year forget 75% of the content covered in a course.

15. T F Active learning requires more preparation by the instructor.

Active learning

Responding to the knowledge explosion by talking faster or packing more facts into the same fixed course and curriculum will not work. Teaching all the content is not the same as having students learn all the content. Take out your college transcript and see if you agree that what the memory retains after a few years is fairly small. I don't remember even *taking* some courses that appear on my transcript much less what was in them. Same with some of the books on my shelves. My marginal notes prove I have read them, but I have no memory of having done so. This is not unusual. On average, students after one year can forget more than half and perhaps two-thirds of the content covered in a course.

The wisdom of the Lakota bears reflection: "Tell me, and I'll listen. Show me, and I'll understand. Involve me, and I'll learn." Psychological investigations yield similar conclusions: many people retain only about 10% of what they hear and up to 90% of what they say and do. Also, the average person can hold only 5-7 bits of information in memory at one time, but acting on that information in some way better ensures it will be saved to long

> The sort of teaching we propose requires that we encourage active learning and that we become knowledgeable about the ways in which our students hear, understand, interpret, and integrate ideas.
>
> *American Association of Colleges Task Group on General Education*

term memory. Active learning works on these principles. Active learning basically means doing something with knowledge, processing it in some way for better understanding and retention.[1]

> Tell me, and I'll listen. Show me, and I'll understand. Involve me, and I'll learn.

This is not to say that lecture is a waste of effort. An enthusiastic and organized lecturer can synthesize and present large bodies of information while modeling thinking and problem solving skills. For conveying factual information to a large number of interested and motivated people, lecture is efficient (though, again, retention of that information may be a problem). If students can be taught and motivated to be active listeners, to participate in a silent dialogue with the lecturer, and to take notes that are more than transcription, students can move beyond understanding to analysis, synthesis, and evaluation.[2]

> Learning is not a spectator sport.
>
> *Chickering and Gamson, 1987*

But for the average lecturer and listener, it is hard to keep attention high for 50 minutes. Breaking a lecture into three or four segments and then pausing for one or two minutes between each segment can help to alleviate that limitation. If at 15–20 minutes into a lecture and then again at 30–35 minutes, an instructor pauses two minutes to allow students to process what they heard — through note reviews, one-minute essays, exchange of notes, group discussion, etc. — student performance can be significantly better on free-recall quizzes and comprehensive tests, enough for up to two letter grades difference.[3]

In lecture, note-taking too can be a mechanical process in which information passes through the ear to the hand without passing through the brain. Going to class and taking notes are important, but one study suggests that neither is as important as processing the knowledge, which in this case, requires reviewing the notes before taking an exam. Students who did not go to class and studied someone else's notes did better than those who went to class and took the notes but did not review them.[4]

Thus, at the level of recognition and recall, active learning facilitates learning. Nonetheless, even if we grant this and perhaps recognize the possibility that because of technological and social innovations students now have different learning styles than we did in school, it is still easy to sympathize with critics such as P. F. Kluge who lament the need for "Sesame Street techniques" in higher education. I, for one, do not believe all active learning strategies enhance higher order thinking or even lower level learning. As a participant I have been frustrated at development programs that involve collaborative learning activities where the ignorant exchange their ignorance while the program coordinator smiles approvingly at the intensity of the mindless interaction. It is easy to forget that encouraging students to be active is a method to reach a goal, not the goal itself. On the other hand, well-planned, guided activities can help students to move beyond memorization toward more holistic processing of ideas. Active learning improves retention and also can stimulate thinking at higher levels.

A reason for this is that knowledge is not the same as information. Information can be transmitted, knowledge cannot. Knowledge requires learners to process information: to infer, interpret data according to previous experiences, create relationships, fit information into existing cognitive structures. Knowledge is generated, not transmitted, by the learner in response to what is transmitted. Thus, for example, to encourage critical thinking, questioning rather than lecturing may be more effective, for the questions stimulate mental activity whereas the answers may bring it to rest.[5] If students are more than auditors (i.e., if they become involved in case studies, role plays, Socratic questioning, oral reports, and group problem solving), they are more likely to be motivated to higher order thinking and to a greater awareness of attitudes and values.[6]

> We say we want students to *analyze* (a critical thinking objective), but our testing largely asks them to memorize. We say that we want our students to be able to *evaluate*, but many of us construct our tests out of multiple choice and true/false questions. We say that we want them to be able to *articulate* positions and *dispute* arguments, but we require them to write very little... and we lecture to them day in and day out when they sit doing what? Analyzing? Articulating? Thinking critically? Not so that you'd notice.
>
> *Marshall W. Gregory*

Another point to remember is that active learning is not just, or even primarily, a classroom strategy. Homework should be active learning. Reading, for instance, can be just as passive as listening to a lecture. The crucial difference is not whether information is taken in orally or visually. Active reading means that students mark main ideas in the books, take time to notice structure, analyze the arguments, write in questions and objections, and propose alternative solutions. Directed reading assignments that prompt students to perform these activities allow class time to be spent not on disseminating information but on applying and analyzing the information gleaned from reading.

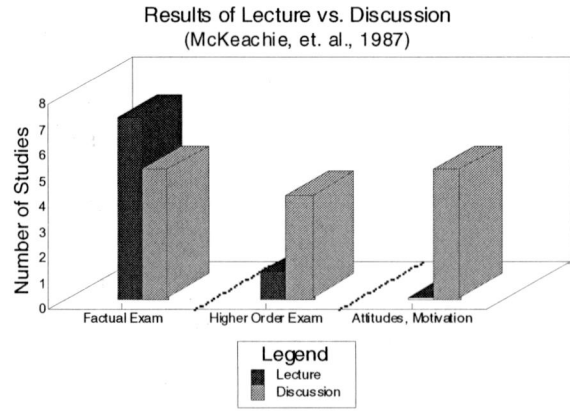

Reprinted with permission by Pearson Custom Publishing. Results of Lecture vs. Discussion (graph). In: Feldman K, Paulsen M. Teaching and Learning in the College Classroom, Second Edition. Upper Saddle River, New Jersey: Pearson Education; 1998.

Active learning also helps create the learner-centered environment that many educational organizations, including the American Association of Colleges of Pharmacy (AACP), have recommended to prepare students to become life-long learners. The "sage on the stage" paradigm of education needs to be supplemented by a model of learning in which the learner is the center of the educational process and the instructor is a mentor or facilitator, the "guide on the side." Self-directed learners do not walk out of classrooms in which for three hours a week for 16 weeks students have been an audience for the performer in the front of the room.

Active learning is a broad term that can be applied to a number of teaching strategies. It can refer to brief classroom techniques for engaging students, (i.e., a think/pair/share or fishbowl to facilitate discussion), a brain dump to focus students on a topic and to assess their current level of understanding, or a directed reading to encourage comprehension of reading assignments (see the "Menu of Active Learning Strategies" at the end of this chapter for explanations of these terms). It also can refer to

> ...A major responsibility of pharmacy educators is to shift the burden of learning from the teacher to the student. The transition from a dependent learner to an independent learner must occur as the student progresses through the pharmacy curriculum. ...Teaching must be achieved through educational processes which involve students as active learners. Teachers must view themselves as coaches and facilitators rather than merely as providers and interpreters of information.
>
> *Background Paper II*
> *Commission to Implement Change*
> *in Pharmaceutical Education*

more general methodologies such as collaborative learning or Socratic dialogue. Of particular interest here is active learning that constitutes practice of clearly defined ability outcomes, or components of those outcomes: case studies, simulations, role plays, supervised professional responsibilities — activities that can be performed in the classroom, as homework, and in the clinic and other experiential settings. These "practice opportunities" are extremely helpful in developing the abilities students need for success within their profession.

Active Learning in Pharmacy Education

Pharmacy educators and practitioners have been alert in recognizing first that the evolving health care environment (e.g., cost containment; home-care, self-care, ambulatory care; drug and dosage forms innovations; computer technology; health care reform; mail order) is changing the current practice of pharmacy, and secondly that such changes in practice will necessitate changes in educational methodologies.[7] AACP Background Paper II envisioned the change this way:

> ...A major responsibility of pharmacy educators is to shift the burden of learning from the teacher to the student. The transition from a dependent learner to an independent learner must occur as the student progresses through the pharmacy curriculum. ... Teaching must be achieved through educational processes which involve students as active learners. Teachers must view themselves as coaches and facilitators rather than merely as providers and interpreters of information.[8]

Along these lines, Strand and Morley, for instance, conclude that new educational goals require new educational models. The psychometric model, anchored in empiricism and didacticism, assumes the student to be a passive object in the learning process. The epistemological model assumes the student is an active organizer and constructor of knowledge. In contemporary pharmacy education, didacticism and the memorization of facts remain important, but a "systematic, cognitively-based approach to problem solving is a 'natural' consequence of a curriculum designed to produce critical thinkers."[9] Content-based, instructor-centered methods of education are effective for conveying extraordinary amounts of information fairly economically to a large number of students while providing "safe" roles for both instructors and students. However, to develop future practitioners skilled in problem-solving and critical reasoning, a student-centered approach is probably more effective.[10]

Collaborative Learning

Collaborative learning is an umbrella term for a variety of group approaches to education that include cooperative learning, problem-centered instruction, Guided Design, case studies, peer teaching, simulations, and learning communities.[11] An important benefit of collaborative learning in pharmacy education is that it helps prepare students for a work force in which group dynamics and interpersonal skills are becoming more essential in the health professions.

In group learning students teach one another and take responsibility for one another's learning. This is effective for the learner because the tutor often understands better than the teacher the tutored student's thinking processes and vocabulary. The student is more likely to ask questions and challenge a peer tutor than he or she would an instructor. Even more beneficial is that the tutor comes away with a better grasp of the material because, as all instructors know, teaching is one of the best forms of learning. Students also recognize from group learning that there are multiple perspectives to issues and alternate ways of organizing and processing knowledge. This type of interaction encourages development of critical thinking skills.

The formation of groups depends upon the purpose for creating the groups in the first place. Some instructors allow students to self-select, often resulting in friends gravitating together. This has an advantage of immediate cohesiveness, but a problem is that friends are less likely to challenge one another or to report a group member whose behavior seriously jeopardizes the group's chances of success. Also, a significant benefit of group learning is for students to work productively with people they don't know well or perhaps even don't like. Some instructors assign students to groups based upon abilities, grouping weaker students with stronger; this can cause the weaker students to feel self-conscious and the more gifted students to feel exploited. Generally, random selection of group members may be the best approach.

Case Studies

Within pharmacy education, case studies and problem-based learning are popular active learning strategies to teach thinking and problem-solving skills. Though often cases are used within problem-based learning (PBL), a distinction between the two is that traditional case studies usually are preceded by didactic transmission of knowledge, which is then applied to a particular case, whereas PBL is a more radical educational strategy requiring students to find and organize the knowledge they will need to analyze the case. Cases can be short classroom activities, projects, or the entire subject matter of a course.

Case studies are useful tools but as with all tools, students should be taught how to use them.[12] Faculty, particularly in the early years, should begin with simple cases. Objectives should be clear; the process should be rehearsed, and criteria for successful analysis should be explained. At first, it may be a good idea to limit discussion to isolated individual components of the case. As the students become familiar with the process, they can be given cases that involve greater complexity and ambiguity, that have multiple answers or no clear-cut correct answers. The scope can be broadened to include sociological, political, economic, and ethical issues. Videotapes, simulations, and participation by real patients increase interest levels.

Problem-Based Learning

The desire to transform students from dependent to independent learners is a motive for the development of problem-solving curricula in medical education and more recently in pharmacy education (see Chapter 3 above for a discussion of PBL).

Problem-based learning is offered in a variety of different formats that configure various combinations of case studies, simulations, collaborative learning, and experiential training. There are many ways these programs could be categorized. One way is to place them on a continuum between a "guided discovery approach" and an "open discovery approach."[13] Guided discovery is highly structured with outcomes prepared in advance for students, though the students may not know what they are. Open discovery requires more self-directedness for students, who are responsible for creating the outcomes they hope to achieve as well as the strategies for achieving them.

Guided Design as a method to promote higher level cognitive practices has been employed in courses in Principles of Pharmacy Practice, Non-Prescription Drugs, Clinical Research and Self-Care Pharmacy Practice.[14]

Problem-solving approaches closer to the models of Woods and McMaster are reported as being effective for teaching Pharmacotherapy,[15] Pharmaceutical Care,[16] Pharmaceutics,[17] Clinical Pharmacokinetics,[18] Externships/Clerkships,[19] and Alcohol and Drug Abuse.[20] For low-cost, individualized, and self-paced instruction, computers can be an effective tool to help students develop problem-solving skills.[21]

Role-playing and Simulations

Role playing and simulations exploit the problem-solving practice required by case studies but in addition to intellectual challenges they also offer multidimensional experiences in dealing with the psychological and emotional reactions that attend decision making within realistic contexts. Even though they know the simulations are not real, students experience some of the frustration, anger, and satisfaction that they would if they were in an actual social situation. These insights into human reality cannot be taught through traditional classroom strategies. Simulations differ from experiential training in that they offer "safe" environments where mistakes have less consequential effects. Learning about bankruptcy by playing Monopoly© is less risky than investing $40,000 in the market. Recommending amoxicillin/clavulanate to treat an upper respiratory infection in a patient who previously experienced an anaphylactic reaction to penicillin has fewer repercussions in a classroom than in a clinic. Experience may be the best teacher, but it also can be the worst teacher if your mistake results in serious harm to yourself or others. Nonetheless, for students prepared to move beyond simulations, carefully structured and monitored experiential educational programs are invaluable for learning how to function effectively in a practice setting.

Writing as Active Learning

> "Patient has been married twice, but denies any other serious illnesses."
> "Patient experiences difficulty swallowing tires easily."
> "Patient referred to hospital by private physician with green stools."
>
> *Cory D. Fox, The Write Stuff:*
> *A Grammatical Overview of Medical Records*

As these chart notes demonstrate, writing in the health professions sometimes falls a little short in clarity and accuracy. Clearly, learning to write is important for pharmacy students entering a career that is evolving toward a practice that requires more communication and interpersonal skills. But writing, besides being a desired ability outcome in and of itself, is also a strategy for developing other general and professional abilities. In other words, students should learn to write and also "write to learn."[22] Most of the problems we have in writing do not come from an inability to use commas or to avoid sentence fragments. What makes writing difficult is that it requires us to clarify our ideas, to organize them effectively, to analyze them, to provide evidence for them, to judge whether our arguments and the arguments of others are valid and convincing. This is critical thinking. One of the best ways to teach critical thinking within a pharmacy curriculum is to incorporate more written assignments that require a rigorous, thoughtful engagement with concepts, issues, and practices relevant to the profession. The rationale and some strategies for this are discussed at length in Chapter 7.

Experiential Education/Laboratories

Pharmacy education has the advantage of being practice-based, which means it has a strong tradition of laboratory and experiential learning, highly effective active learning strategies that existed long before "active learning" became pedagogical buzz words. The manipulating, measuring, observing, conjecturing, and testing that occur in investigative laboratories clarify understanding and sharpen thinking abilities. Experiential education as a capstone experience allows students to integrate their learning at a practice site, and more recently the inclusion of early practice experiences into pharmacy curricula has demonstrated the applicability of classroom knowledge to professional settings. In addition, the idea of experiential education has broadened so that knowledge and skills as well as attitudes and values are its targets. Service learning, for instance, is a form of experiential learning that seeks to promote student empathy by situating them in caring relationships with the elderly, infirmed, homeless, abused, impoverished, mentally ill, and other disadvantaged persons in the community. Of course to maximize the benefits of experiential education, it should be structured with stated outcomes, clear criteria, and ongoing formative feedback from a preceptor.

Active Learning: Problem or Opportunity?

Active learning is not without its liabilities.[23] Active learning initially does require more preparation by the instructor, particularly if the instructor has been using canned lectures that change little over the semesters. And obviously some active learning strategies are less effective or practical in large classes. Creative instructors usually can find and adapt active learning strategies to the size of their classes, but still, smaller classes do allow for more individualized instruction and more opportunities for feedback. Thus, active learning may require additional financial and human resources. Learning styles differ among individuals, and some students actually prefer the anonymity of passive learning, but most students do not resist active learning strategies once they have participated in well-planned and effective activities. Finally, depending on how it is done, employment of active learning strategies can result in less coverage of content during the class presentation, as doing takes more time than hearing. In a content-laden discipline such as pharmacy, this is a real issue that each instructor must wrestle with.

> There are two kinds of teachers: the kind that fill you with so much quail shot that you can't move, and the kind that just gives you a little prod behind and you jump to the skies.
>
> *Robert Frost*

Regarding content, two arguments in support of active learning can be given. Some instructors believe that hearing less but learning better is a worthwhile trade-off if students also can be given the self-learning skills to find and understand new material on their own. This is particularly true in a curriculum designed to teach critical thinking. Linda Salamon's evaluation of the pharmacy curriculum of the mid 1980s points up this tension between the paradigms of learning as storage and learning as growth:

> The problem is that it [the curriculum] offers too much knowledge with too little attention to how that knowledge has been created and what methods and styles of inquiry have led to its creation.[24]

The poet Robert Frost agrees that information presented as endless agglomerations of discrete and unrelated facts can stymie rather than stimulate student learning: "There are two kinds of teachers: the kind that fill you with so much quail shot that you can't move, and the kind that just gives you a little prod behind and you jump to the skies."

A second argument is that active learning can actually result in learning more content. This argument challenges two assumptions. First, the assumption that coverage of content means the same as learning of content. Have instructors reached their educational outcomes if they ignore students' raised hands because they feel pressured to get to the last sentence of their lecture notes? Coverage of 100% of the material with student understanding and retention of 50% is less efficient than coverage of 80% of the material if students can both retain and understand 70–80%.

A second assumption is that students can learn content only from what they hear in the classroom. If students are expected to learn facts from reading and homework assignments prior to coming to class, the classroom time normally devoted to transmission of facts would be available for activities that broaden and deepen their understanding. Practice of abilities rather than just transmission of knowledge can become the goal of classroom instruction. Having picked up the content through assigned directed readings, for instance, students in the classroom can then apply that knowledge as they participate in simulations, role plays, and discussions that are oriented toward thinking, communicating, and ethical decision making within professional contexts.

Regardless, most agree that with the knowledge explosion, doubling information in some disciplines every decade or less, covering all the content in any three semester-hour course will require lecturers and listeners to have fast forward buttons surgically implanted. It is time to consider alternatives.

Adoption of critical thinking as a course outcome requires selection of teaching strategies that will promote the learning and practice of critical thinking. The conclusion sounds obvious, but unfortunately the mismatch between desired outcomes and teaching methods occurs too frequently.

> We say we want students to *analyze* (a critical thinking objective), but our testing largely asks them to memorize. We say that we want our students to be able to *evaluate*, but many of us construct our tests out of multiple choice and true/false questions. We say that we want them to be able to *articulate* positions and *dispute* arguments, but we require them to write very little … and we lecture to them day in and day out when they sit doing what? Analyzing? Articulating? Thinking critically? Not so that you'd notice.[25]

Lighting Fires or Filling Buckets

W.B. Yeats' view of education is right: Education is not filling a bucket but lighting a fire. Education is not just cognitive activity. It is imaginative, emotional, even visceral and involves motivation, ideals, goals, values, attitudes. Boring a hole into someone's head and pouring in facts is an educational paradigm that cannot survive in the information age regardless of how much content there is to learn. Lighting the fire in students means helping them develop the knowledge, skills, and desire to learn. It means inspiring them through example and getting them involved in their learning. Graduates, even of pharmacy schools, are not filled buckets and never can be. Our teaching strategies must reflect that. If lighting a fire is our goal—the development of the skills and habits and values of lifelong learning—then we need to have "matches" that work.

> Education is not filling a bucket but lighting a fire.
>
> *W.B. Yeats*

Quiz Answers

Oh yes, the quiz. Did you take the pop quiz at the beginning of this chapter? If so, did it have any effect on how you read the chapter? Did you try to find out during the reading whether or not your answers were correct? A quiz such as this can serve as a way to direct student reading. When students are given questions before a reading assignment, they are alerted to key points and are encouraged to form hypotheses, which will be tested during the reading. The reading becomes more interesting because of the intellectual challenge. To avoid mechanical, rote responses, ask some questions that are not easily picked out by skimming or that require higher order thinking. In addition to questions answered in the reading, require students to make inferences or draw conclusions. The quiz format allows for self-satisfaction when right answers are given, and encourages students to formulate arguments when their responses do not agree with the answers in the reading. In short, the quiz can help turn reading into an imagined dialogue.

Holding a Cat by the Tale?

That chapter title is inspired by Mark Twain, who was a bit skeptical of some educational enterprises, as evidenced by his cynical witticism: "First God made fools. That was for practice. Then he made school boards." But as a son of the "Show Me State" of Missouri, he did place high value on experiential learning: "The person that had took a bull by the tail once had learnt sixty or seventy times as much as a person that hadn't..." No matter how good the lecture about grabbing a bull's tail, it cannot compete with the active learning experience. And along the same lines: "A person that started in to carry a cat home by the tail was getting knowledge that was always going to be useful to him, and warn't ever going to grow dim or doubtful."

> A person that started in to carry a cat home by the tail was getting knowledge that was always going to be useful to him, and warn't ever going to grow dim or doubtful.
>
> Mark Twain

In short, holding a cat by the tale, like other active learning experiences, provides you with long-lasting practical knowledge you can achieve in no other way.

Following is a menu of simple active learning strategies that can be adapted for pharmacy education. These strategies exemplify a wide range of possibilities, some being comparatively simple techniques that can be incorporated fairly easily, others perhaps requiring complete revision of a course or even a curriculum. Additional information about many of these and other acting learning strategies can be found in:

Angelo TA and Cross KP. *Classroom assessment techniques: a handbook for college teachers*, 2nd ed. San Francisco: Jossey-Bass, 1993.

Bean J. *Engaging ideas: the professor's guide to integrating writing, critical thinking, and active learning in the classroom.* San Francisco: Jossey-Bass Publishers, 1996.

Bonwell C and Eison J. *Active learning: creating excitement in the classroom.* ASHE-ERIC Higher Education Report No. 1. Washington, D.C.: The George Washington University, 1991.

Gibbs G. *Discussion with more students. Developing teaching: Teaching more students.* Oxford: The Polytechnics and Colleges Funding Council, 1992.

Karre I. *Busy, noisy and powerfully effective: cooperative learning in the college classroom.* Stillwater, OK: New Forums Press, 1993.

Meyers C and Jones TB. *Promoting active learning: strategies for the college classroom.* San Francisco: Jossey-Bass, 1993.

Silberman M. *Active earning: 101 strategies to teach any subject.* Boston: Allyn and Bacon, 1996.

Sutherland T and Bonwell CC, eds. *Using active learning in college classes: a range of options for faculty.* San Francisco, CA: Jossey-Bass, 1996.

A Menu of Active Learning Strategies

Writing Activities

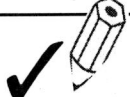

Minute Essay (Microtheme)
At the beginning, middle, or end of the class, ask students to write down what is unclear, what questions they have, what the main point of the lecture was, what objections they may have to the ideas being presented, or what was the most beneficial or insightful part of class. Limit the writing to a short period of time and/or have the students write their responses on a 3-by-5 card. In large classes, sample the responses and provide feedback during the next class period.

Brain Dump
A short writing exercise in which students write down everything they know about an announced topic. This stimulates student attention and provides feedback to the instructor about the students' knowledge base.

Directed Reading
Create a set of questions for students to answer after they have completed a reading assignment so that they are prepared for a discussion of the subject matter in class. This allows class to be focused on analysis and synthesis of information rather than communication of facts.

As an alternative, ask students to write three questions they formulated based on the reading assignment or to find arguments that were incomplete or questionable.

Admission ticket
Require submission of a previously assigned writing project (such as a directed reading) to get into class.

Summary of Summaries
Students write a 2–3 page summary of an assigned reading and exchange summaries. Each student then writes a 1-paragraph summary of the other person's 2–3 page summary.

Journals
Require students to keep course journals in which they record chapter summaries, homework questions, and individual insights and questions about course material. Provide feedback at least three times a semester. In large classes, be selective in the reading of journal entries. Ask students to mark their three best entries; read those and three others at random.

Question Box
Students have the opportunity to drop off written questions to which the instructor can respond in class or privately.

Writing Assignments to Simulate Future Activities
Create and model writing assignments which will prepare students in the practice of pharmacy (e.g., patient counseling, defense of papers/presentations, analysis of journal articles, abstracts of articles, analysis of current newspaper/magazine articles, preparation of research proposals, summaries of current drug information, and letters of application).

Collaborative Learning

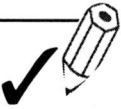

Team Activities

In large classes, create teams of four or five students. Periodically stop the lecture to ask the students to perform group tasks, such as solve a problem, pose a question, make cognitive maps, create outlines, paraphrase the lecture to each other, create test sample questions, and identify basic principles of the day's topic.

Think/Pair/Share

Ask students to write for a few minutes on an assigned topic or question. Then they spend another few minutes discussing with a partner, comparing and testing their ideas. Finally, the groups report their ideas to the entire class. Students thus have time to think their thoughts through and to obtain private feedback before responding to the entire class.

Pyramid

Version of think/pair/share in which students begin to tackle a problem individually, then in twos, then fours, and so on until the whole class shares their ideas.

Notes Exchange

In the middle of a lecture, pause to allow students to exchange and compare class notes so that students can see another perspective or another way of arranging material.

Peer Teaching

Have students master different parts of an assignment and then teach one another the sections they have learned.

One-on-One

In groups of two, one student presents a sustained explanation of point, question, or difficulty to another student whose role it is to keep the other student focused. After the assigned amount of time, the students exchange roles.

Paraphrase to Different Audiences

To encourage students to develop perspective and to improve their interpersonal and communications skills, ask them to explain the same topic or process to two different audiences. The assignment can be written, performed within groups, or performed in front of the class.

Collaborative Writing

In large classes form teams of four and assign four essays to each team. One person takes responsibility for writing the essay and the other three take responsibility for providing feedback to the writer about content, style, and mechanics. Each person has a turn as writer. Students evaluate the essay and the group performance of each individual.

Assessment as Learning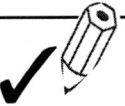

Self-assessment Check-sheets
Along with an assignment, hand out the criteria by which the assignments will be judged and ask the students to assess how well they met the criteria. This process allows students to correct any errors or omissions in the first attempt.

Peer Assessments
Students evaluate one another's work according to explicit criteria which requires students to identify the elements that make the work successful. This evaluation process not only provides feedback to the peer but also enables the assessor to improve his or her own performance through a better understanding of the performance criteria.

Construct Assessment Criteria
Ask students as individuals to formulate the criteria with which to assess an assignment they have been given and then to work in groups of two or four to extend and refine the criteria.

Assess Sample Performances with Criteria
Distribute a sample student performance that marginally meets the criteria and ask students to assess it using the criteria. Discuss the responses. Repeat the process first with an excellent performance and then with a weak performance. This provides students with a better understanding of what constitutes good practice.

Grading as a Learning Exercise
Grade tests and quizzes in class so that students can get feedback on their performance and on ways to improve. Then ask the students to revise or repeat the performance.

Lecture Alternatives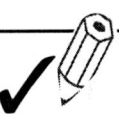

Socratic Questioning
Rather than tell students the solutions, ask questions that require them to work through the solutions themselves, probing their assumptions, questioning their data, and explaining their thought processes. In the process students learn how to evaluate evidence.

Simulations
Students act out social or professional situations, demonstrating the knowledge, skills, attitudes, and values required to perform well in those situations.

Role Playing
Students assume an identity and try to reconstruct how that person would act in a particular situation. Other students provide feedback. Have the students switch roles and/or interact with different audiences, explaining a drug recommendation to a doctor, nurse, patient, and family member.

Lecture Alternatives (Continued)

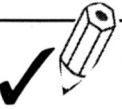

"Physical" Education
Involve students by having them use their bodies. Force position-taking by votes with raised hands or by movement to one side of the room or the other. Ask students to act out complex or abstract ideas such as molecular bonding.

Intentional Errors
Make an intentional error in class. Continue with the error until students question and correct you. For students used to passive learning, you may travel well into absurdity before they will express their confusion.

Pause
Stop the lecture for three minutes so students can review their notes and formulate questions or ideas.

Fishbowl
Four to eight students conduct a discussion while the remaining students outside the "fishbowl" can listen but not comment. One chair is left vacant for an "outsider" to become a participant if he or she feels compelled. The "forbidden fruit" phenomenon stimulates participation.

Case Studies
Create scenarios that require to integrate their skills to solve problems that relate to course material.

Evaluation Grids
Ask the students to create tables in which they list the positive and negative features of an idea, action, or thing. Compare with another student and/or discuss in class.

Defining Features Grids
Ask the students to create tables in which they compare and contrast ideas and objects by identifying the presence or absence of features. Compare with another student and/or discuss in class.

Student Presentations
As individuals or groups, have students research, organize, and communicate their ideas on an assigned topic to the class. For sophisticated presentations, require multimedia and computer components.

Posters
As individuals or groups, have students research, organize, and communicate their ideas on an assigned topic in poster format.

Lecture Alternatives (Continued)

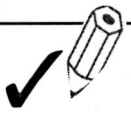

Problem-Based Learning
Present a problem, allowing students to determine what they must know to solve the problem, and provide mentoring as students find, comprehend, analyze, and synthesize the material in order to solve the problem.

Debates
For controversial topics, ask students to defend a position using arguments that are logical, developed, complete, and convincing.

Experiential Learning
Provide opportunities to do something with their knowledge in a real-life situation.

Games
Design friendly competitions to promote learning of material that is mostly facts or terminology. *Jeopardy*© is a popular format.

Questions for Reflection

1. To what extent does your teaching focus on content, abilities, and/or students?
2. To what extent are you currently employing active learning in classroom and experiential settings?
3. Which of the active learning strategies listed could most easily be incorporated into your teaching?
4. Which active learning strategies would most enhance the learning of your students?
5. What could you plan to transform a 50-minute lecture class into an active learning session employing three to four activities that require students to put their knowledge to work in the practice of abilities?
6. What are the barriers for including more active learning in your teaching?
7. How can the impediments be addressed?

Notes

1. A good overview of the philosophy, goals, and methods of active learning can be found in Bonwell CC, Eison AJ. Active learning: creating excitement in the classroom, ASHE-ERIC Higher Education Report No. 1. Washington DC: George Washington University, 1991. Since Bonwell was director of the Teaching and Learning Center at the St. Louis College of Pharmacy when the first draft of this chapter was written, it will be easy to find his influence here.
2. See Bonwell CC. The enhanced lecture: a resource book for faculty. Cape Girardeau, MO: The Center for Teaching and Learning, Southeast Missouri State University, 1991.
3. Ruhl KL, Hughes CA, Schloss PJ. Using the pause procedure to enhance lecture recall. Teacher Educ Special Educ 1987;10:14-8.
4. Kiewra KA, DuBois NF, Christian D, McShane A, Meyerhoffer M, Roskelley D. Note-taking functions and techniques. J Educ Psychol 1991;83:240-5.

5. King A. Inquiry as a tool in critical thinking. In Halpern DF, ed. Changing college classrooms. San Francisco: Jossey-Bass, 1994:13-38.
6. McKeachie WJ, Pintrich PR, Lin Y, Smith DAF. Teaching and learning in the college classroom. Ann Arbor: University of Michigan, 1986.
7. Chalmers RK. Pharmacy education strategy: the solution is in the problem. Am J Pharm Educ 1988;52:388-93.
8. American Association of Colleges of Pharmacy. Background Paper II: Entry-Level, Curricular Outcomes, Curricular Content and Educational Process [1990]. Commission to Implement Change in Pharmaceutical Education. Am J Pharm Educ 1993;57:377-85.
9. Strand LM, Morley PC. Evolving health care systems: academic implications for teaching methodologies with emphasis on administration and practice. Am J Pharm Educ 1987;51:402-6.
10. Strand LM, Morley PC. A problem-based student-centered approach to pharmacy education. Am J Pharm Educ 1987;51:75-79. Also see Odedina, FT, Clemmons, CD, Dukes, N. Mulifaceted active learning approach to teaching pharmacy health care and behavior. Am J Pharm Educ 2000;65:276-83.
11. For an overview of descriptions of collaborative learning, its implementation, and its assessment, see Goodsell AS, Maher MR, Tinto V, Smith BL, McGregor J, eds. Collaborative learning: a sourcebook for higher education. University Park, PA: National Center on Postsecondary Education, 1992. See also Cooper JL, Robinson P, McKinney M, Cooperative Learning in the Classroom. In Halpern DF, ed. Changing college classrooms: new teaching and learning strategies for an increasingly complex world, ed. San Francisco: Jossey-Bass, 1994. Davidson N, Worsham T, eds. Enhancing thinking through cooperative learning. New York: Teachers College Press, 1992. For an application of group learning to case studies in pharmacy, see Sims PJ. Utilizing the peer group method with case studies to teach pharmacokinetics. Am J Pharm Educ 1994;58:73-7.
12. See Hawthorne EM. Case study and critical thinking. Issues and Inquiry in Coll Learning and Teach 1991;15:60-1. Hafler JP. Case writing: case writers' perspectives, in Boud D, Feletti G, eds. The challenge of problem based learning. New York: St. Martin's Press, 1991:150-8.
13. Swanson DB, Case SM, van der Vleuten CPM. Strategies for student assessment. In Boud D, Feletti G, eds. The challenge of problem based learning. New York: St. Martin's Press, 1991: 260-73.
14. Experiments with Guided Design in pharmacy include: Wales CE, Nardi AH. It takes thinking to produce a scholar. Am J Pharm Educ 1988;52:385-8; Chalmers RK. Pharmacy education strategy: the solution is in the problem. Amer J Pharm Educ 1988;52:388-93. Pawlak SM. Development and validation of guided design scenarios for problem-solving instruction. Am J Pharm Educ 1989;53:7-16. Meyer SP, Popovich NG. Experience and observations about the guided design instructional methodology. Am J Pharm Educ 1990;54:35-9. Lush RM III, McAuley JM, Kroboth PD. Experimental design for clinical research: a student-centered problem-based approach. Am J Pharm Educ 1993;57:39-43. Newton GD, Tracy TS, Popovich NG, The development and implementation of an integrating pharmacy practice laboratory. Am J Pharm Educ 1990;4:138-45. Newton GD, Popovich NG, Lehman JD. Development and evaluation of computer-assisted guided design for problem-solving instruction in self-care pharmacy practice. Am J Pharm Educ 1991;55:301-10.
15. Winslade N. Large group problem-based learning: a revision from traditional to pharmaceutical care-based therapeutics. Am J Pharm Educ 1994;58:64-73. Fisher RC. The potential for problem-based learning in pharmacy education: a clinical therapeutics course in diabetes. Am J Pharm Educ 1994;58:183-9. Delafuente JC, Munyer TO, Angaran DM, Doering PL. A problem solving active-learning course in pharmacotherapy. Am J Pharm Educ 1994;58(1):61-4.

16. Sibbald D. Innovative, problem-based, pharmaceutical care courses for self-medication. Am J Pharm Educ 1998;62:109-119. Catney C M, Currie J D. Implementing problem-based learning with WWW support in an introductory pharmaceutical care course. Am J Pharm Educ 1999;63:97-104.

17. Haworth, LS, Eriksen, SP, Chmait, SH, et al. A problem-based learning case study approach to pharmaceutics: faculty and student perspectives. Am J Pharm Educ 1998;62:398-405. Culbertson VL, Kale M, Jarvi EJ. Problem-based learning: a tutorial model incorporating pharmaceutical diagnosis. Am J Pharm Educ 1997;61:18-26.

18. Mehvar, R. Development and evaluation of quasi problem-based objective-driven learning strategy in introductory and clinical pharmacokinetic courses. Am J Pharm Educ 1999;7:17-27.

19. Raisch DW, Holdsworth MT, Mann PL, Kabat, H. Incorporating problem-based, student-centered learning into pharmacy externship rotations. Am J Pharm Educ 1995;59:265-72. Culbertson VL, Kale M, Jarvi, EJ. Problem-based learning: a tutorial model incorporating pharmaceutical diagnosis. Am J Pharm Educ 1997;61:18-26. Nii LJ, Chin AA. Comparative trial of problem-based learning versus didactic lectures on clerkship performance. Am J Pharm Educ 1996;60(2):162-4. Kane MP, Briceland LL, Hamilton RA. Solving drug-related problems in the professional experience program. Am J Pharm Educ 1993;57:347-51.

20. Busto U, Knight K, Janecek E, Isaac P, Parker K. A problem-based learning course for pharmacy students on alcohol and psychoactive substance abuse disorders. Am J Pharm Educ 1994;58:55-60.

21. Boh LE, Pitterle ME, Wiederholt JB, Tyler LS. Development and application of a computer simulation program to enhance the clinical problem-solving skills of students. Am J Pharm Educ 1987;51:253-61. Newton GD, Popovich NG, Lehman JD. Development and evaluation of computer-assisted guided design for problem-solving instruction in self-care pharmacy practice. Am J Pharm Educ 1991;55:301-10. Catney CM, Currie JD. Implementing problem-based learning with WWW support in an introductory pharmaceutical care course. Am J Pharm Educ 1999:63 97-104. Rhodes DG. A practical approach to problem-based learning: simple technology makes PBL accessible. Am J Pharm Educ 1999;63:410-4. Abate MA, Meyer-Stout PJ, Stamatakis MK, Gannett PM, Dunsworth TS, Nardi AH. Development and evaluation of computerized problem-based learning cases emphasizing basic sciences concepts. Am J Pharm Educ 2000;64:74-82. Monaghan MS, Vanderbush RE, McKay AB, Gardner SF, Schneider EF. A computerized database approach to enhance critical thinking. J Pharm Teach 1999;7:35-50. Haworth IS, Bolger MB, Eriksen SP. The use of computer-based case studies in a problem-solving curriculum. Am J Pharm Educ 1997;61:97-102.

22. Volumes of literature relating to writing to learn are nicely summarized in Holiday-Goodman M, Lively BT. Writing across the curriculum for colleges of pharmacy: a source book. Toledo, OH: University of Toledo, Toledo College of Pharmacy and American Association of Colleges of Pharmacy, 1992.

23. Barriers to implementation of active learning are summarized in Charles Bonwell and James Eison, pp. 53-64.

24. Salamon LB. Integrity in the pharmacy curriculum. Am J Pharm Educ 1985;49:362.

25. Gregory MW. Critical thinking and liberal education. Perspectives 1988;18:15-6.

Chapter 6: Using Assessment to Structure Learning: Putting It All Together

> One of the striking things about the responses to our survey was how much attention was given to assessment of learning outcomes and how little to teaching students how to achieve them.
>
> *"Student Learning Outcomes,"* Alverno College

An orientation to teaching means getting one's bearings—recognizing where we are, where we want to go, and what the principal landmarks are along the way. A fundamental starting point is the recognition that teaching is a profession based on fiduciary relationships: instructors' primary obligation is to the success of their students. Caring practitioners require caring teachers and mentors. Second, the practice of pharmaceutical care requires an expanded vision of professional education. Professional *training* remains important in the preparation of a pharmacist who delivers pharmaceutical care, but renewed emphasis is also needed on professional education. Even further, teaching general abilities within professional pharmacy contexts is more likely to produce practitioners who are critical thinkers and problems solvers, effective communicators, and astute ethical decision makers. The adoption of a "learning paradigm" helps instructors to re-vision their teaching so as to be better prepared to enable students to achieve these desired outcomes. Recognizing that students should not passively absorb delivered content but should actively construct knowledge, instructors can organize teaching experiences that are student-oriented and ability-centered. Active learning strategies directed toward critical thinking and problem-solving can help students to attain the knowledge, skills, and attitudes they need to be successful. It is time now to try to pull everything together through assessment.

Assessment has preoccupied higher education in the United States and elsewhere for the past 15–20 years. Colleges and universities are under pressure to demonstrate to constituencies that their missions are being accomplished. This accountability is particularly pressing with a perception of a growing disconnect between student performance and grades, a traditional means for demonstrating effectiveness. But the motivation for assessment is more than a defensive response to external calls for accountability. The more successful schools have embraced assessment as a means to enhance effectiveness of institutions and students, to find out what is working and what is not in order to make structured changes in programs and curricula. Across the country a wide variety of such successful outcomes assessment initiatives have been implemented.[1]

Educational assessment takes many forms and can be classified in a number of ways. The assessment can be of institutions or individuals. Institutional assessment can evaluate programs, divisions, curricula, co-curricular efforts, aggregate student performance, teaching, and so on. Individual teachers and of course individual students can be assessed. For such assessment investigators can analyze empirical data (e.g., test results, summative testing, grades, portfolios, licensure rates, employment data, direct observation, peer reviews, awards, and student publications) and attitudinal data (course evaluations, focus groups, exit interviews, alumni surveys, and reflection essays).

Nonetheless, the assessment movement makes some faculty groan. Some view assessment as an intrusion into one's classroom or clinic, a potential violation of academic freedom, or an impossible task for which they are not methodologically prepared and for which they have little interest and time. Particularly when imposed, assessment appears irrelevant to teaching and learning, especially if faculty believe that it is impossible to assess what is really important in an education.

Here we focus exclusively on assessment of individual student academic performance based upon empirical evidence of student work. What is proposed here is an assessment process that originates with faculty and is controlled by faculty, a process that is part of the teaching and learning process, not an addendum to it. Among the many reasons to assess students, two are most relevant here: 1) to find out what students have learned, and 2) to help them learn better. One assessment approach that undertakes such efforts is "Ability-Based Education" (ABE).[2]

Often assessment is thought to come at the end of the educational process, as an evaluation of what learning has taken place. Putting assessment at the *beginning* of the educational process can help to clarify what is to be taught, when it should be taught, how it should be taught, who should teach it, and how it can be determined whether learning has taken place. A difference is that in ABE assessment is built into the educational process from the beginning as a measurement of what learning has occurred, and also as a tool for facilitating learning. In other words, ABE is built upon the concept of Assessment-as-Learning, in which summative assessment has an important role, but priority is placed on formative assessment.[3]

Simply, ABE establishes educational goals and then designs a pedagogy, a curriculum, and assessment strategies that support those goals. Ability outcomes differ from some other educational outcomes goals by focusing on what students should be able to do as a result of instruction. What students can do, their abilities, do not refer to discrete, atomistic "objectives" but to complex integrations of knowledge, skills, attitudes, habits, and values. These outcome abilities drive the instructional and assessment processes, and they shape both the structure of the curriculum and the institution's organization, policies, and practices.

Ability-based educational assessment can be examined in two dimensions: at the course and at the curriculum levels. ABE entails the redesigning of individual courses and the teaching strategies by which they are taught, but it also involves the creation of a curricular plan that interconnects those courses and gives the curriculum coherence by structuring it around the attainment of specific ability outcomes. When ability-based processes are implemented at both the course and curricular levels, students can progress through a curriculum in which the development of their abilities is the organizing principle. Effectively implemented, ABE has the possibility of transforming pharmacy education so as to better prepare students for the mission of rendering pharmaceutical care.[4] This chapter examines ABE at the course level, suggesting how assessment can help to structure learning experiences in the classroom and clinic.[5]

Ability-based Principles at the Course Level

Though there are other approaches, the method presented here for creating a course structured on ability-based principles involves four steps: identifying ability outcomes, creating opportunities for students to practice the abilities, establishing clear criteria so students can determine strengths and weaknesses in their performance of the abilities, and providing assessment feedback from self, peers, and experts. So, the four steps are:

1. Ability outcomes
2. Practice opportunities for students to practice the abilities
3. Clear criteria that describe what constitutes good performance
4. Assessment feedback about how to do better

Though listed sequentially here, the steps are recursive in nature. For instance, in order to design practice opportunities, one must have some concept of criteria for successful performance, but after observing the performance, faculty and students almost invariably extend and refine the criteria that had been established prior to performance. In other words, the four steps are ongoing and cyclic instead of linear.

Step 1: Ability Outcomes

An ability outcome states what the students will be able to do as a result of instruction. The underlying philosophy is that whereas knowledge is an extremely important and necessary goal of the instructional process, knowledge alone is not sufficient. What students are able to do with their knowledge becomes the basis for evaluation of their success. Such a focus on abilities, on what students can do, does not undervalue content or knowledge, as some faculty sometimes fear. One cannot, for instance, think critically or monitor pharmacotherapy without a solid knowledge base. But an ability-based approach does require students eventually to move beyond the lower levels of Bloom's Taxonomy (recall, comprehension) as they use their knowledge base to perform complex disciplinary tasks.

Terminology varies.[6] For some educators, "objectives," "competencies," and "ability outcomes" are used interchangeably. Here we will make some distinctions regarding these types of outcomes, but there are some similarities. All outcomes normally should be written to describe what the student will be able to do as a result of instruction, not what the course will do or what the instructor hopes to do. For instance, an outcome is not "introduce students to principles of therapeutics," but "apply therapeutic principles in the monitoring of therapies." Outcomes also are different from course activities. What students do in the course (i.e., practice opportunities) are methods for achieving outcomes, not the outcomes themselves. For example, "the student will gather materials for a report on chemical dependency" or "students will work in groups to create a presentation on AIDS" are course activities, not outcomes. What they are trying to achieve through those assignments are the outcomes.

However, not everything that students do is classified as an ability. An ability is different from objectives in that it is more complex and holistic. Unlike objectives that are usually more specific, atomistic, and discrete, an ability is an integration of knowledge, skills, and attitudes/habits/values.[7] For instance, two objectives might be, "at the end of this lecture the student will be able to identify three causes of pneumonia" and "at the end of this lecture the student will be able to calculate creatinine clearance." The first objective is useful knowledge, and the second is an important skill, but neither would be classified under this system as an ability. If one were to ask why the student should know about the causes of pneumonia or how to calculate creatinine clearance, it would be clear that these objectives are components of more comprehensive abilities, such as "educating patients and health care professionals" or "recommending drug therapy." Thus objectives often are one of the three components (knowledge, skills, attitudes/habits/values) that together make up an outcome ability. For instance:

Ability Outcome	1. Counsel patients on Antimicrobial drug therapies	
Objectives	A. Acquire antimicrobial knowledge base, etc.	(Knowledge)
	B. Adapt communication to audience, etc.	(Skills)
	C. Exhibit empathy, etc.	(Attitudes)

Objectives are an important instructional tool for clarifying learning expectations for the student, helping the instructor create an educational plan to achieve the objectives, and providing a basis for assessment. Linking objectives to ability outcomes provides a clearer understanding of why the objectives are being taught and how they are interrelated.

The crucial distinction is that abilities are multidimensional, requiring for their mastery a variety of educational experiences. Within a medical framework, Epstein and Hundert suggest the levels of integration that are necessary in order to become competent in one's profession:

> Competence builds on a foundation of basic clinical skills, scientific knowledge, and moral development. It includes a cognitive function—acquiring and using knowledge to solve real-life problems; an integrative function—using biomedical and psychosocial data in clinical reasoning; a relational function—communicating effectively with patients and colleagues; and an affective/moral function—the willingness, patience, and emotional awareness to use these skills judiciously and humanely. Competence depends on habits of mind, including attentiveness, critical curiosity, self-awareness, and presence. Professional competence is developmental, impermanent, and context-dependent.[8]

Types and Levels of Ability Outcomes

It is important to recognize that ability outcomes can be written to reflect varying levels and expectations of student achievement. Outcomes that must be achieved by the end of curriculum are "terminal outcomes." But during the course of instruction, "enabling" or "developing" outcome statements can be constructed to specify what the student must achieve at the end of a course or even of an assignment. A hierarchy of ability outcomes might extend from assignments to profession as follows:

- Interprofessional (e.g., IOM outcomes)
- Profession
- Institutions (general and professional outcomes)
- Colleges of pharmacy (general and professional outcomes)
- Divisions/departments
- Individual courses
- Assignments

Not all of these levels are applied at every institution, but what is important to recognize is that the lower levels of ability outcome statements make more specific and limit the more general outcome statements that come before them. In other words, all the levels are articulated and integrated.

For instance, professional outcomes define the abilities a student must exhibit upon graduation to enter a profession. The AACP Center for Advancement of Pharmaceutical Education (CAPE) Outcomes, for example, describe three broad practice functions for which entry level practitioners should be prepared.

- Pharmaceutical care
- Systems Management
- Public Health

As terminal outcomes, or what is expected to be demonstrated upon graduation, the CAPE Outcomes do not provide levels of performance to be achieved during specific intervals within the curriculum; i.e., they do not provide enabling ability outcomes to be employed at the division or course levels.

The CAPE Outcomes provide a framework for abilities required to practice pharmacy in the beginning of the 21st century, which are meant to be adapted by faculty at their own institutions, according to their institution's philosophy and educational values. The values, traditions, goals, and resources of each institution influence how the faculty at that institution define the terminal college ability outcomes a graduate must demonstrate. Common ability outcomes for colleges include general outcomes:

College Outcomes	General Outcomes Think critically Communicate effectively Resolve ethical dilemmas Professional Outcomes Provide pharmaceutical care Manage systems Collaborate in interprofessional teams

In some university settings, the university may have developed general ability outcomes for the entire institution, with the expectation that colleges of the university would develop corresponding outcome statements for their students.

University Outcome	The student shall find, understand, analyze, evaluate, and synthesize information and make informed, rational, and responsible decisions.
Professional or College Outcome	The student shall interpret and evaluate pharmaceutical data and related information needed to prevent or resolve medication-related problems or to respond to information requests.

At some institutions, in order to provide additional guidance in the teaching and assessing of abilities, individual departments develop divisional outcome statements that further break down the college/program outcomes. Thus a Pharmacy Practice Department might address a college outcome of "provide pharmaceutical care" by adopting divisional ability outcomes such as these:

Pharmacy Practice Division Outcomes	Select/recommend drug therapy. Evaluate drug therapy. Monitor drug therapy. Communicate with patients, care-givers, and health professionals. Educate patients, care-givers, and health professionals. Collaborate with health care professionals.

The Pharmacy Administration Department would flesh out divisional outcomes that relate to the management function.

Course ability outcomes derive from and make even more specific the college or divisional outcomes. A course ability outcome specifies how this course will attempt to help achieve a part of the college/divisional outcome ability and designates the level at which the ability is expected to be demonstrated in this course.

Divisional Outcome	Evaluate the appropriateness of patient-specific therapies.
Course Outcome	Evaluate at an intermediate level the appropriateness of uncomplicated patient-specific antimicrobial therapies.

Objectives or Abilities?

Can you distinguish which of the following are objectives and which are ability outcome statements?

1. Select/Recommend appropriate drug therapy for specific patients.
2. Identify the signs and symptoms associated with Parkinson's disease.
3. Monitor for efficacy, adverse effects and toxicity relating to aminoglycoside therapy.
4. Educate patients and health care professionals regarding antibiotic therapy used to treat this patient's urinary tract infection.
5. Calculate creatinine clearance using the Cockroft and Gault equation.
6. Recommend appropriate treatment for a patient presenting with hypertensive emergency.
7. Demonstrate the steps involved in phagocytosis.
8. Understand the pharmacology (i.e., mechanism of action, adverse effects, drug interactions) of the oral sulfonylureas.
9. Demonstrate confidence in communication with physicians and other health care professionals.
10. Use organizational behavior concepts and frameworks to identify and analyze the variables that can influence employees' job satisfaction, absenteeism, productivity, and turnover.

Answers

Numbers 2, 7, and 8 are *knowledge* objectives. They require understanding of facts. The verbs "identify," "demonstrate," and "understand" suggest lower order thinking is required. Asking "why" students would "identify signs and symptoms" or "demonstrate the steps in phagocytosis" might lead to formulation of an ability outcome statement.

Number 9 also is an *attitudinal* objective. "Communicate effectively with physicians and health care providers" would be a program ability outcome statement. One facet of such communication is having confidence.

Number 5 is a *skills* objective. One reason a person might calculate creatinine clearance is to "recommend drug therapy"—an ability outcome.

Numbers 1, 3, 4, and 6 are course ability outcomes. The performance of each requires an integration of knowledge skills, and attitudes, including some of the objectives appearing on this list. Number 1 is a college ability outcome; 3, 4, 6 are course ability outcomes because they are more specific and limited.

Number 10 is unclear whether it is an ability outcome or objective. It should be rewritten so that students understand more clearly what is expected of them.

It should be clear that no course outcome (other than perhaps the outcomes for advanced practice experiences) should be an exact copy of a college, division, or CAPE outcome, for that would imply that that one course would result in attainment of the ability at the professional entry-level. No one course alone can enable students to achieve a college outcome, much less a CAPE outcome. Abilities are developed gradually, in incremental fashion, over the years of a curriculum. The course outcome above limits the division outcome by concentrating only on antimicrobial therapy and by focusing on uncomplicated cases. Other courses in the curriculum would adopt course outcomes that cover other types of therapy and would pitch their instruction at different levels. Courses that come earlier in the curriculum would operate at a more basic level whereas later courses would require students to perform at a professional entry level. All the course outcomes in this series, when taken together, would equal the college or program outcome. In particular, it would be unlikely that any course/practice experience prior to the last year of the curriculum would have an ability outcome that is identical to any CAPE outcome (or any college outcome) unless it is true that within that capstone course or practice experience students will demonstrate that ability outcome to a degree indicative of an entry-level practitioner.

Integrating Ability Outcomes

There are many different ways to organize outcome statements, and faculty should design a format that corresponds to their goals, for the formulation of outcomes plays a significant role in what is taught and assessed in the classroom and practice site. A positive innovation in the 2004 CAPE Outcomes is the attempt to integrate general and professional outcomes within courses and experiential activities. In the CAPE Outcomes, the description of "Pharmaceutical care" is as follows:

> Provide pharmaceutical care in cooperation with patients, prescribers, and other members of an interprofessional health care team based upon sound therapeutic principles and evidence-based data, taking into account relevant legal, ethical, social, economic, and professional issues, emerging technologies, and evolving biomedical, sociobehavioral, and clinical sciences that may impact therapeutic outcomes.

And the subdivisions make it clear that thinking, communicating, ethical decision-making, and self learning need to be taught within professional contexts: "Design, implement, monitor, evaluate, and adjust pharmaceutical care plans that are patient-specific and evidence-based"; "communicate and collaborate with prescribers, patients, care givers, and other involved health care providers to engender a team approach to patient care." In other words, thinking, for example, can be explicitly taught within practice functions, such as selecting/recommending drug therapy or assessing disease states, if the following outcome criteria are adopted in courses such as pathophysiology or therapeutics:

- Describes the general thinking/decision-making process
- Uses a framework in thinking/decision-making
- Identifies, interprets, analyzes, evaluates, and synthesizes information to make rational, responsible decisions
- Collaborates with others involved in decision-making process
- Makes complex decisions in a variety of environments

And similarly, self learning can be shown to be an important component of abilities such as monitoring drug therapy if the following outcome criteria are integrated into professional functions:

- Identifies various tools and methods of learning and demonstrates personal responsibility for achieving ability outcomes.
- Selects own approach to learning and shows how and why it works best for him/her.
- Uses perceptive and insightful self-assessment and feedback from experts and peers to drive learning and improve personal performance and abilities.
- Applies self-assessment and feedback from others to enhance learning and ability achievement in a collaborative setting.
- Uses metacognitive strategies to conduct continual self-assessment of self-learning in order to develop and enact a plan to improve performance thus ensuring ongoing professional competency.[9]

An ability-based approach is most effective when faculty review their courses, determine what they want their students to be able to do as a result of instruction, and integrate the desired knowledge, attitudes, and skills into course ability outcomes that are clearly stated on a syllabus. Often this process is transformative and heuristic as the instructor begins to explore possibilities that have not been taught or assessed before. For example, to which commonly practiced professional abilities could you add criteria such as:

- listens actively to patients and/or caregivers
- exhibits empathy and compassion
- accepts a fiduciary responsibility for patient well-being
- treats all socio-economic classes and races equally
- respects decisions made by competent patients and caregivers
- exhibits conscientious approach to patient care (e.g. diligent follow-up, comprehensive monitoring)
- displays confidence in one's competence as a health care provider
- displays assertiveness in management of drug therapy
- accepts constructive criticism

Rethinking one's goals (i.e., asking "which attitudes or values are needed for this ability") may lead to the inclusion of material that might not otherwise have been covered, (e.g, ethical dimensions embedded within one's discipline, empathic responses in patient communication, or mutual respect in collaborative efforts between health care professionals). In this way an ability-based approach leads to an integration of professional and general educational goals, and to the development of a better-prepared practitioner.

Thus the reason for carefully crafting ability outcome statements is to inform students about what they need to accomplish in the classroom or experiential environment, but also to decide what should be taught and how the learning activities should be structured. In a course on herbal products, if the outcomes are "Be familiar with the botanical classification into which plants are divided" or "Know the source, active ingredient, and physiological effects for at least one drug derived from each of the structural classes presented," the expectations for the students mainly are lower level thinking skills as identified in Bloom's taxonomy, requiring mainly reading and listening. But if ability outcomes are created so that students must "Find, comprehend, analyze, and evaluate information relating to the most commonly used natural products" and "Communicate effectively with patients regarding the use of natural products," then the instructor must reorganize the course to create opportunities for students to practice these higher level abilities, which is Step 2 in this ability-based approach.[10]

Steps for Creating Ability Outcomes

- Make a list (brainstorm) of what you think is important in your course.
- Review the list. See what goes together, what is repetitive, what can be combined, whether one statement is a subset of another. Group them and create an outline.
- Determine if what you expect your students to know from your course is related to what you expect your students to be able to do, and vice versa.
- See if you can distinguish in your list which statements pertain to knowledge, skills, or attitudes/habits/values.
- Try to integrate the objectives regarding knowledge, skills, and attitudes into a statement about ability outcomes. (Sometimes, you can determine your ability outcomes by asking why you want your students to know or be able to do something.) Normally, two to four ability outcomes are the most you might want to include in each course because there may not be enough time for the practice opportunities and assessment feedback needed to develop each ability.
- Determine if general abilities (thinking, communication, ethical decision-making) are sufficiently integrated with your professional goals.
- Review your list to see if anything is missing. Often this process is heuristic, a mechanism for discovering ideas you did not think of in the brainstorming stage. For instance, asking "what attitudes" are needed for this ability may lead you to include material into the course that you might not have otherwise, for instance a case analysis that raises issues relating to empathy or fiduciary obligations to patients.
- Relate your course outcome abilities to college or program outcome abilities, if they exist. The course outcomes should breakdown the college/program outcomes. Rather than repeating the college/program outcomes, course outcomes should be an adaptation of the college/program outcomes relevant to the content and level of this particular course.
- Clearly state the course ability outcomes on the syllabus so that students know exactly what they must do to be successful in the course.

Step 2: Practice Opportunities

A premise of ABE is that abilities must be practiced in order to be achieved. In other words, active learning is built into the logic of ABE. It is highly unlikely that students who are exposed only to traditional didactic forms of instruction will develop abilities such as critical thinking as a result of that instruction.[11] In an ability-based approach, the course outcomes determine the teaching strategies that are employed. Lecture is a powerful tool for communicating knowledge to a large number of students, but it is much less effective for developing skills, attitudes, and values. Thus ABE requires multiple teaching strategies (including lecture), for unless students are given frequent opportunities to practice course ability outcomes—whether the abilities are thinking, communication, or implementation of a drug therapy plan—they are unlikely to improve as much.

The practice of abilities can take place in homework, in classroom activities, or in experiential settings. A practice of the course outcome could be an essay, presentation, project, role-play, simulation, debate, case study, exam, clinical activity, creation of "a peripheral brain" or personal pharmacotherapeutic resource, service learning activity, laboratory experiment, directed reading, etc. Again, such practices are designed to reinforce acquired knowledge through the use of it. Some assignments can be created to help students learn specific knowledge, skills, or attitudes that make up an ability outcome. Other assignments can require students to practice the integration of the appropriate knowledge, skills, and attitudes. What is important is that students are given ample opportunities to practice at the appropriate curriculum level.

If students see the connection between course ability outcomes and practice opportunities, they are more likely to improve; therefore, the syllabus should clearly relate the practice opportunities (assignments, projects, course activities, etc.) to the appropriate course outcomes. Also, the practice opportunities and the assessments should overlap. If the students practice abilities during the course but are graded upon other criteria such as acquisition of data (or vice versa if they are presented with information but are required to demonstrate abilities at testing time), they may lose confidence in the approach. More productive would be to weight the practice activities such that the grade attached to the activity is proportionate to the importance of the outcome. Frequent practice opportunities can present challenges to instructors of large classes, but note that not all practice activities must be graded. In fact, Assessment-as-Learning should involve some "risk-free" practice. Individual or group feedback to such practice will likely result in better performance at the time of summative testing or "validation," at which point students are required to demonstrate they can meet the expected outcome.

Steps for Creating Practice Opportunities

- Review the course ability outcomes. Determine teaching strategies that will allow students to practice those abilities or their associated learning objectives.
- Ensure that the learning strategies promote the achievement of the abilities you have chosen as course outcomes, that is, that they give students sufficient opportunities to practice the abilities.
- Design multiple assignments that provide sufficient opportunities for students to practice the ability outcomes at varying levels of difficulty.
- In the syllabus, clearly relate the practice opportunities (assignments, projects, course activities) to the appropriate course outcomes.
- Note that not all practice activities must be graded. Formative assessment (Assessment-as-Learning) can involve some "risk-free" practice.
- Weight the practice activities such that the grade attached to the activity is proportionate to the importance of the outcome or to the attainment of the outcome (e.g., if written communication is a primary ability outcome, the course grade weighting should reflect that).

Step 3: Performance Criteria

In ability outcomes education, the basis for assessment is performance criteria—descriptions of the behaviors or actions the students must demonstrate if they are to be capable of performing the outcomes. The criteria clearly describe for the student 1) what he or she must do to successfully practice the ability, and 2) the guidelines by which it will be determined how well he or she performs. Performance criteria allow the instructor to gather observable, documented evidence regarding outcome attainment.

Performance criteria are related to a "performance" (i.e., a practice of the course ability outcome, such as an essay, home work assignment, presentation, project, role-play, laboratory experiment, OSCE, in-basket, drug information paper, or clinical activity).

Criteria are not directions for the assignment or algorithms for the performance of the task. Criteria are the measurements by which instructors and students can assess how well students are doing in the practice of the course outcomes and more importantly, another tool for students to learn to improve their performance. Performance criteria are often difficult to construct, for instructors may never have been required to make explicit their assumptions about what constitutes good performance in their disciplines. They can recognize it but not easily verbalize it. But novices, the students, lack that background, that tacit recognition of competent performance, and so they sometimes become frustrated when they receive a "C" on what they had thought had been an excellent performance. They may have been unable to do what was expected of them, but they did not know what the expectations were. By knowing explicitly and up-front what constitutes good performance, students can better prepare to meet the course outcomes.

It is also important for faculty to determine at what level of performance (e.g., beginning, intermediate, advanced) students must perform in this course, and to write criteria to reflect that appropriate level of performance. Given the place of the course within the curriculum, faculty may decide to emphasize or ignore specific performance criteria, knowing that deeper or more complete coverage of the ability will occur later in the curriculum.

Stating the criteria often is not sufficient. Students must understand them. Until students have direct experience with the criteria, until they have applied them in their own work and have seen concrete examples of successful and unsuccessful practice plotted against them, the criteria may not be as particularly helpful for them. For instance, for the ability outcome, "monitor for expected therapeutic outcomes and potential adverse effects with selected drug therapy," one criterion is "establishes intervals and frequencies for monitoring parameters." The criterion is clearly stated, but until students see the statement applied to actual performances, they may honestly believe they are achieving the criterion when they are missing key components. Assessment feedback provides this clarification, and it is also helpful to devise exercises so that students better comprehend the basis for what constitutes good performance.

For instance, students can empirically "discover" criteria if they are given examples of performances at various levels of proficiency and are asked, as individuals and in groups, to rank them and then to determine the basis for their rankings. One method is for the instructor to give an example of a moderately successful performance of a case analysis and to ask the students 1) to assess it as individuals, 2) to share their assessments with another student, 3) and explain their assessments in group discussion. In the process students, perhaps without knowing it, are empirically creating criteria for successful

Outcome: Find, analyze, evaluate, and communicate drug information.

Practice Opportunity
Find and read an article in a popular journal that discusses Rogaine. In a 3–5 page essay written for a lay audience, summarize, analyze, and evaluate the article so that your readers can make informed decisions about the drug.

Performance Criteria:
1. Accurately summarizes reading
   - Clearly states the main idea/argument
   - States major supporting ideas/arguments accurately
2. Analyzes facts, ideas, and issues,
   - Provides necessary background
   - Determines accuracy, significance, fairness, logic
3. Evaluates facts, ideas, and issues
   - Clearly articulates a judgment about value or correctness
   - Provides basis or criteria for the judgment
   - Provides evidence for the judgment
4. Communicates information effectively
   - Adapts communication to audience
   - Presents information in a clear, organized manner

Sample Criteria

Evaluate patient-specific drug therapy and therapeutic problems.

Assess appropriateness of current therapy
- Critically analyze indication(s) for each medication
- Identify contraindications for therapy
- Identify untreated problems
- Determine efficacy of current agents
- Determine need for preventative medicine

Assess compliance
- Inquire about patient's pattern of medication use (methods of administration, missed doses)
- Verify patient understanding of indications for medications
- Verify patient understanding of drug regimens
- Compare patient's understanding of drug indication and regimen with patient profile and label directions
- Check refill records
- Check compliance with clinic/office appointments

Recognize adverse drug reactions
- Classify adverse effects according to outcome (i.e. fatal, life-threatening)
- Explain, when asked, the significance and mechanism of ADRs

Recognize drug interactions
- Classify drug interactions (p'kinetic vs. p'dynamic)
- Explain, when asked, the clinical significance and mechanism of interaction(s)

Developing Abilities Across Levels

Valuing and Ethical Decision-Making
Displays the habits, attitudes, values, and ethical decision-making required to render pharmaceutical care

Level 1
Develops an understanding and framework for valuing and ethical decision-making
- Understands and articulates the values and principles of professionalism (i.e., empathy, compassion, honesty, integrity, accountability, altruism, service-orientation, trustworthiness, competency, desire for learning, confidence, tolerance, cooperation, leadership, autonomy, justice)
- Understands and articulates the behaviors of professionalism
- Understands and articulates the values and principles of pharmaceutical care
- Articulates one's personal values and how they influence the practice of pharmacy and ethical decision making
- Uses an ethical decision-making rubric to apply basic ethical theories and principles

Level 2
Independently practices and evaluates valuing and ethical decision making within the classroom and introductory practice experiences (IPEs)
- Identifies and analyzes ethical dilemmas that arise in professional contexts
- Identifies and analyzes the role of personal values in professional interactions
- Makes and defends ethical decisions in case studies
- Demonstrates values and principles implicit in pharmaceutical care at IPE sites

Level 3
Collaborates in ethical decision-making
- Respects the values, opinions, and arguments of others in the group
- Defends one's position in a logical, nonconfrontational manner
- Demonstrates willingness to compromise without compromising his/her own integrity

Level 4
Exhibits professionalism and ethical decision-making at practice sites
- Maintains professionalism at practice sites
  - Displays a service orientation
  - Establishes fiduciary relationships with patients
  - Exhibits conscience and trustworthiness
  - Displays accountability for his/her work
  - Displays leadership
  - Commits to self-improvement
- Makes and defends informed ethical decisions in professional settings

performance. The process can be repeated with a weak performance and again with an excellent case analysis. Through discussion the instructor can modify, adapt, and formalize the criteria the students created until the criteria approximate those created by the instructor. Finally, the instructor can distribute these revised criteria to students and ask them one more time to assess the same performance they evaluated without criteria. What usually results is better understanding of what constitutes good practice of an ability, and greater accuracy and consistency in assessment. Such exercises allow students to understand and internalize the criteria, rather than simply to depend upon them as check-lists or algorithms.

The process also works well for instructors to achieve consistency in assessment, both in one instructor's evaluation of several individual students in a class and in multiple instructors' assessment of the same student. It is not uncommon in a group of 15 instructors for their assessment of the same student's work to range in grades from "A" to "D." Without a shared vision of what constitutes good performance, instructors prioritize, valorize, or ignore different aspects of a student's work and come up with valid, justifiable but wide ranging conclusions. Assessment that is anchored to specific, clearly defined criteria removes some of the subjectivity and randomness. In workshops settings, participants who undertake the assessment tasks described in the previous paragraph are likely at the end of the process to come within a half letter grade of one another in their assessment of student work.

Sometimes, it is assumed that some components of an ability are ineffable: They cannot even be taught much less assessed. That may be true. Habits, values, and attitudes do present particular challenges for the instructor. Nonetheless, some strategies can be developed. In a service learning course, for instance, students can be asked to explore their attitudes toward care and empathy as they keep a journal of weekly reflections about their service activities. Grading such subjective reflections is rife with difficulties, but creation of objective criteria can provide integrity to the process.

Journal Criteria

1. Observe
   - Accurately and vividly record objective observations of your site experiences (events, peoples, actions, setting).
2. Record your response
   - Convincingly record your subjective responses to your service experiences (your thoughts, emotions, values, and judgments).
3. Analyze/Evaluate
   - Find insights, patterns, structure, categories, meanings, causes, effects, and relationships in what you observed and reflected upon.
   - Evaluate facts, inferences, and your personal responses, determining the correctness or relative suitability of actions, beliefs, systems, and attitudes.
4. Plan
   - Identify the knowledge, skills, attitudes, and resources needed to be successful.
   - Devise strategies to procure the necessary knowledge, skills, attitudes, resources
   - Create specific action plans to improve service, both your own and the agency's.
   - Modify actions plans as necessary.

Students are assessed not on how much they "care" or how empathic they are in their weekly encounters with persons in need, but on their ability to observe, reflect, analyze, and plan. In the process of observing, reflecting, analyzing, and planning, it is hoped that they become better able to put themselves in the place of another person, but there is no guarantee that they will. At least the journals will have helped them develop the cognitive abilities to know what it means to demonstrate empathy if not the inclination to be empathic. With appropriate criteria, it is a risk worth taking.

Detailing criteria can be time-consuming and frustrating.[12] As experts in their disciplines, instructors have internalized but not always made explicit for themselves or others what constitutes good performance of abilities. They can immediately recognize good performance, but a comprehensive description of good performance is not so easily achieved. The frustration can be increased when faculty discover that refinement of criteria is usually an iterative, ongoing process. Often when faculty assess student work, they find that students met all the criteria but still did not perform well. When assessing students in cooperation with other faculty members, they sometimes discover aspects of performance they had not considered. Criteria may need to be modified or new criteria may need to be inserted. The end result, though, is that continual refinement of criteria provides students with a better picture of what they are supposed to be doing and thereby increases their ability to do it.

Steps for Creating Criteria

- For each course activity, list what knowledge, skills, and attitudes/values/habits must be present for the performance to be judged successful. (This is often difficult to do in that we may never have been required to make explicit our assumptions about what constitutes good performance.)
- If you have them, review assignments you have previously graded. Make explicit the reasons you assigned the grades that you did. Compare your grading criteria to those of your colleagues. Determine if your grading criteria accurately reflect successful performance of the ability you are hoping students will learn.
- Arrange the criteria into outline format.
- Determine at what levels students must perform in this course (e.g., beginning, intermediate, advanced) or at this particular place in the course. Write the criteria to reflect the appropriate level of performance.
- Clearly write in the syllabus the performance criteria that will be used to assess the performance of the major practice opportunities. If this is cumbersome, state that performance criteria for each assignment will be distributed when the assignment is made.
- Link the course grade directly to achievement of performance criteria. If 90% of the course grade is based upon objective test scores, students will place little value on attainment of abilities.

Step 4: Assessment Feedback

After students 1) have been told what abilities they must demonstrate to pass the course, 2) have been given opportunities to practice the abilities, and 3) have been told what constitutes good practice, they need 4) to receive assessment feedback regarding how well they have performed.

Summative assessment is the type many of us are most familiar with. Summative assessment occurs at the end of instruction. Its purpose is to evaluate, to determine rank, to give a score, to justify progression or matriculation. A summative assessment certifies achievement, the way a final exam measures a student's performance in a course.

In formative assessment, on the other hand, the primary motivation is to enhance student learning. Unlike summative assessment that occurs at the end of instruction, formative assessment is concurrent with learning; in fact, it is part of the learning process itself. In formative assessment students are asked to demonstrate what they have learned and then are given feedback about how they can do better. When such assessment is performed regularly and consistently, it is labeled, "Assessment-as-Learning." Summative assessment measures progress; Assessment-as-Learning enables progress.

Assessment-as-Learning

ABE is structured on the philosophy of Assessment-as-Learning.[13] That is, assessment is a continuous, formative part of the learning process. Assessment feedback after performances enables students to improve their abilities in the next performance. Assessment is an important teaching tool, not merely a method by which to demonstrate to accrediting agencies and other external constituencies that the academic program is sound, although ability-based processes can perform that function also.

Some feedback is more helpful than others. Feedback can be simply a response in terms of Lykert scales, check marks, pluses and minuses, smiley faces, or numerical scores from 1–10. Written comments such as "nice job," or "needs work" or "try harder" give an indication of value but provide little direction for the student.

Assessment feedback is most helpful when it is

- Criteria-referenced
- Evidence-based

"Criteria-referenced" means that specific, public performance criteria provide the framework for the feedback given. "Evidence-based" means that the feedback cites elements of the student's performance apropos the criteria. That is, the assessment is based upon achievement of the criteria (criteria-referenced), and specific examples from the student performance are used to acknowledge strengths and to suggest ways to improve (evidence-based). Evidence-based, criteria-referenced assessment conducted by instructors, students, and peers, enables:

- A better student understanding of good performance in assignments
- Opportunity for students to improve prior to submission/performance
- Identification of specific student strengths/weaknesses
- Directed and specific feedback to enhance student performance
- A basis for consistency in evaluation from student to student and instructor to instructor
- Collection of specific evidence regarding student learning for program improvement

If at the time a practice opportunity is assigned criteria are provided along with the directions for the assignment, students have a better understanding of what they are supposed to do. If students are asked to recommend drug therapy for a particular case, they may correctly identify the drug, dose, and route, but they might not justify their selection because they did not know that justification was expected. If the students are given the following criteria for the ability to select/recommend, their performance will improve almost automatically:

Select and recommend drug therapy for specific disease states.

- Includes plan for existing therapy
- Identifies correct new drug therapy (i.e., drug, dose, route, frequency and duration) based on guidelines and primary literature
- Justifies the complete drug therapy plan based on drug- and patient-specific data
- Incorporates results from the primary literature when justifying therapy decisions
- Briefly explains why other drugs were not chosen based on the evidence

Because, as we have seen, performance criteria describe the knowledge, skills, and attitudes that delineate good practice of an ability, the criteria are the basis for providing assessment feedback. It is helpful for instructors to reproduce the criteria and use the page as a feedback form. The instructor can mark on the form after each criterion to what degree the student achieved that expectation.

Again, the feedback is not limited to a numerical score or a pithy summary comment. Rather, the feedback consists of explicit, concrete descriptions of 1) what was successful and why, and 2) what behaviors need to be improved and how. The assessor cites examples from the performance that justify the assessment made and provide suggestions on how to improve. In other words, the feedback not only is criteria-referenced but also evidence-based: The feedback is directed toward the student's actual performance, as it is now and as it might become.

An instructor does not need to assess every criterion in every practice opportunity. Some assignments can be constructed to emphasize particular criteria, so that students can learn in a step-wise fashion or so that students can work on criteria they had not met on previous practice opportunities. In this assessment form for written communication, for instance, the instructor may decide that for this practice opportunity grammar or mechanics is not relevant to his or her goals or the instructor may single out adaptation of language as the only criterion.

Assessment Form: Select/Recommend Drug Therapy

1 Not Acceptable	2 Needs Development	3 Competent Performance	4 Excellent Performance
Generally incomplete or incorrect. Requires frequent & extensive assistance or intervention; facilitator and/or peers must complete sections.	Only partially complete or correct. Requires consistent assistance or intervention; facilitator and/or peer must often assist in selecting/recommending patient cardiovascular therapy and in answering questions.	Generally complete and correct. Requires infrequent assistance or intervention; student is consistently able to select/recommend patient cardiovascular therapy and answer questions without assistance.	Exemplary. Requires rare assistance or intervention; student is able to select/recommend patient cardiovascular therapy and answer questions without assistance. Could be used as a model for best practice/performance.

Performance Criteria	Assessment Score	Evidence
Includes plan for existing therapy		
Identifies correct new drug therapy (i.e., drug, dose, route, frequency and duration) based on guidelines and primary literature. (ex., "Recommend spironolactone 25 mg daily based on RALES trial and recommendations by the ACC/AHA guidelines")		
Justifies the complete drug therapy plan based on drug- and patient-specific data (ex., "starting warfarin at ½ the normal maintenance dose was done b/c patient is also on amiodarone therapy" or "dose of spironolactone was decreased to 25 mg qod because of the rise in serum K to 5.3", or "spironolactone is appropriate in this patient b/c he is currently in class NYHA IV HF and on other standard HF therapy")		
Incorporates results from the primary literature when justifying therapy decisions (ex., "spironolactone is being added b/c of the 30% decrease in overall mortality over a 24 month time period found in the RALES trial, which studied spironolactone vs placebo in NYHA Class IV HF pts already on standard HF therapy".)		
Briefly explains why other drugs were not chosen based on the evidence (ex., "eplerenone was not chosen as the aldosterone antagonist for this pt b/c it has only been studied in patients with HF post MI [not the case in this patient] and is more expensive than spironolactone")		

Written Communication

Criteria	Score	Evidence
Adapts language style, and tone to a specific audience		
Organizes thoughts in logical sequence		
Sufficiently develops ideas with accurate, convincing evidence and examples		
Uses correct grammar and mechanics		
Overall student performance		

Still, such feedback takes time. To facilitate detailed formative feedback, instructors can construct feedback templates to be used in conjunction with assessment feedback forms. After grading student work, instructors often find that students tend to make common mistakes or exhibit similar deficiencies. These instructors find themselves making the same comments to student after student, a time consuming and tedious process. A feedback template is a set of standard feedback responses organized and numbered for easy retrieval. Instead of writing a detailed comment, the instructor can simply insert, for example, "see 1b," where "1b" would be an explanation of a common error made regarding a particular criterion.

The template responses can consist of a sentence or two, or they can extend to paragraphs or even pages. The instructor can provide a mini-lecture as part of the feedback or can include references and page numbers where students can get additional help. This requires additional preparation, of course, but in the long run can be time efficient, for the responses can be used for all the students in this class as well as in subsequent classes. Preparing generic feedback in advance also allows the instructor to check for clarity and to make sure the comments are written with an appropriate tone, one that motivates rather than deflates. If the templates are encoded electronically, links can be provided that take students immediately to supplementary materials that will help them improve their performance. Particularly useful is the implementation of an electronic portfolio system that lists abilities and criteria and allows self and expert assessment feedback that is evidence-based and criteria-referenced.[14]

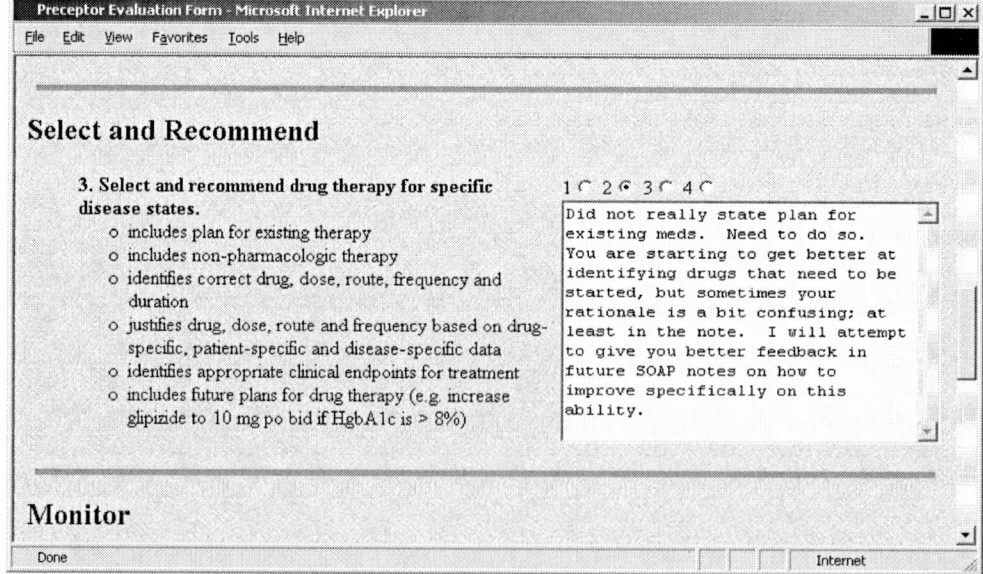

Peer and Self Assessments: Self Learning

Instructor or expert assessment is not the only efficacious method for formative feedback. Self and peer assessments also are useful for developing particular abilities and also for developing self learning and collaboration, both essential for practitioners in health care settings. Being able to identify strength and weaknesses and to identify strategies for improvement undergirds self learning, an invaluable ability in light of the remarkable knowledge explosion. Providing clear and accurate feedback in a diplomatic, encouraging way is crucial for collaboration.

With a list of criteria in hand, students can self assess as they prepare their performance, or afterward, for instance while reviewing a tape of their performance, a portfolio, or a written assignment. If self-assessment sheets are distributed when an assignment is made, students are likely to do better, for they are given a chance to correct the work before the instructor sees it. This is especially true if students must not only evaluate their work according to specific criteria and also provide evidence from their work to justify their evaluations.

If at the time an activity is assigned students are given self-assessment forms to complete, they are unlikely, for instance, to respond "no" to a question that asks, "Did you determine etiologies for each problem when assessing patient-specific states?" More probably, they will go back and fix the problem before completing the assignment. Or, alternatively, if they did not meet the criterion, they might say that they did, for one of two reasons. First, it may be that they did not understand the criterion in the first place and honestly believed they met it. If so, instructor feedback will help them develop a better understanding of expectations. A second reason is that perhaps the students are slacking off and not being entirely honest in their self assessments. This will be less of a problem if students are required to provide specific evidence for their self-assessment.

Eventually, with enough practice and encouragement, students become candid and acknowledge in self-assessments what problems they are still having. They demonstrate a clearer understanding about what constitutes good practice even if they are not yet able entirely to achieve it.

The value of peer assessment is a bit more indirect. Often peer assessment can be time draining and actually counterproductive. If the peers do not understand the material or the criteria, the feedback they are able to give can steer an assessed student in the wrong direction. And even if they are knowledgeable, peers may be unwilling to provide critical feedback for fear of offending the student or negatively influencing his or her grade.

In the early stages of peer assessment, it is probably the peer assessor who benefits most from the process. Criteria, no matter how clearly written, initially will not be completely understood by novices. Self-assessment provides an opportunity to clarify criteria by testing them against concrete cases, but it is difficult to evaluate one's own work—to distinguish what is on the page or in the performance from what is in one's own mind. With a peer, the student knows only what is in the performance or on the page. By analyzing the performance of their fellow students, they themselves understand more clearly, particularly through negative examples, what constitutes successful performance of the ability. They begin to comprehend more fully what the criteria mean, and by providing suggestions for improvement to others, they can improve their own performance of the targeted abilities.

It is important for peers to recognize that their assessments cannot negatively influence a fellow student's grade, but that the assessments can help to improve a student's grade if they provide clear, criteria-based feedback. If students remain reluctant to provide accurate and valuable peer feedback or if they are unmotivated to take the time to do so, an instructor can grade their peer assessments. Structured properly, peer assessment can become a practice opportunity for self-learning and also collaborative learning.

As they become more adept, peer assessors also provide more of a service to the student whose work is being assessed. Sometimes peer feedback can be more useful to a student than expert assessment. Because of common perspectives and similar learning experiences, peers sometimes can understand better fellow students' mistakes or can explain solutions in a shared idiom.

The value of assessment feedback can be lost if students are not given an opportunity to repeat the performance or to perform similar practice opportunities. Ability development requires iterative and recursive practice. If an instructor spends 45 minutes writing comments on a student's drug monograph but then assigns a summative grade and does not give the student an opportunity to rewrite the essay, it is common for a student to look at the grade and not even read the comments, much less try to benefit from them. If, on the other hand, the student must rewrite the monograph (or write another monograph) using the feedback as a guide, the student more likely will try to understand and apply the comments so as to enhance his or her abilities. So, after assessment feedback is given the four-step loop is repeated: a better understanding of the ability outcome, repeated practice, clarification of criteria, and additional suggestions on how to improve.

Effective self and peer assessment does not happen automatically. Faculty should build some time into the course to explain the advantages, difficulties, and methods of self and peer assessments. Students must be taught how and why to assess. Those evaluated must learn to recognize that the feedback they are given is constructive, meant to help them improve. Otherwise the temptation will be for the peer assessors to evaluate too highly and to fail to point out deficiencies, provide evidence for the assessment, and provide suggestions for improvement. If students recognize that peer and self assessment is an opportunity for them to improve their performance (and their grades), they are more likely to assess one another honestly and productively, providing criteria-referenced and evidence-based feedback.

Steps for Creating Assessment Feedback

- Incorporate assessment as part of the learning process, not simply as an after-the-fact measurement of the learning process. That is, provide formative as well as summative assessment.
- For each major course activity, determine appropriate methods of feedback (self, peer, expert). Determine if written or oral feedback (or both) would be most productive.
- Create assessment forms that include the criteria that are needed for students to demonstrate successfully the selected ability outcome at the appropriate level at this stage of the curriculum and course.
- Distribute the assessment forms when the assignment is given so that students can use them to prepare the assignment.
- Require peer/self assessments for some performance/assignments; state this requirement in the syllabus. Design peer assessments that allow the assessors to internalize the criteria and thus to be able to improve their own performance of the ability outcome. Consider making self and peer assessments part of the grade for the assignment.
- Build some time into the course to explain the advantages and difficulties of self and peer assessments. Instruct students on how to assess one another honestly but productively. The assessments themselves can be used as part of the grade for the assignments. State in the syllabus whether or not assessments will be graded.
- In the syllabus, state the assessment processes for each course requirement.

Summary

Assessment can give coherence to a course and a curriculum if clear, specific outcomes are used to determine content, sequence of material, teaching strategies, and evaluation techniques.

Assessment-as-Learning valorizes formative assessment—assessment that does not simply register achievement but helps to promote it.

Ability-based Education uses Assessment-as-Learning principles to help students achieve abilities that are essential for professional practice. As an individual, an instructor can employ ability-based educational approaches to:

- Select and define outcomes that are complex abilities, appropriate to the level of the students
- Structure the course so that practices of the ability outcomes are the major activities
- Construct criteria-referenced assessment tools for each major practice opportunity
- Teach students to self and peer assess
- Enable students to self assess prior to expert assessment
- Require peer assessments that are criteria-referenced and evidence-based
- Provide criteria-referenced evidence-based assessment feedback that enables students to improve.

This has been a far from comprehensive review of educational assessment. Again, this book is meant as an "orientation," not as a complete map of the territory of teaching. For instance, though summative assessment, including assignment of grades, is a very important practical and often perplexing issue for beginning and experienced teachers alike, little mention of it is made here. The goal instead is to provide a model and rationale for assessment that serve as frameworks for faculty as they develop innovative assessment strategies that enable students to become more proficient in their abilities.

The focus here has been on what an individual instructor can do in his or her own course to design educational experiences that promote the development of ability outcomes. Whether or not one's college has adopted an integrated approach to the development of abilities across the curriculum, individual faculty can use ABE strategies to organize their courses and practice experiences according to the development and assessment of ability outcomes.

Exercises

1. Formulate an ability outcome appropriate to a course you are teaching.
2. For that ability outcome, develop two practice opportunities. Be imaginative and unconcerned initially about practicality and resources.
3. For each practice opportunity, develop performance criteria that give a clear picture of what successful practice means (the knowledge, skills, attitudes/habits/values that constitute good practice).
4. For each practice opportunity, choose appropriate methods for assessment feedback. Decide on the mode of feedback (e.g., oral, written, computer-mediated) and the type (self, expert, peer). Create assessment forms that allow for criteria-referenced, evidence-based feedback.

Notes

1. Banta T, Lund J, Black K, Oblander F, eds. Making a difference: outcomes of a decade of assessment in higher education. San Francisco: Jossey-Bass, 1993. Palomba CA, Banta TW. Assessment essentials: planning, implementing and improving assessment in higher education. San Francisco: Jossey-Bass, 1999. A good overview of assessment in pharmacy can be found in Abate MA, Stamatakis MK, Haggett RR. Excellence in curriculum development and assessment. Am J Pharm Educ 2003;67(3):Article 89. For examples of innovative practice of assessment in pharmacy, see Zlatic TD. Redefining a profession: assessment in pharmacy education. In Palumbo C, Banta T, eds. Assessment of student competence in accredited disciplines: illustrative case studies. Sterling, VA: Stylus Publications, 2001.

2. Among the first and most successful proponent of ABE is Alverno College, a women's liberal arts college in Milwaukee. Since the 1960s, Alverno has created much of the vocabulary and many of the processes associated with ABE and now is nationally recognized for its achievement in pedagogical innovation. This discussion, though, is not meant to be an accurate description of the Alverno approach. For that, see Mentkowski M and Associates, Learning that lasts: integrating learning, development, and performance in college and beyond. San Francisco: Jossey-Bass, 2000.

3. Within the assessment field, terminology can vary. Sometimes a distinction is made between "assessment" and "evaluation" or between "formative assessment" and "summative assessment." "Assessment" and "formative assessment" usually refer to feedback meant to improve student performance. "Evaluation" and "summative assessment" normally refer to measurement of students' educational success, such as through test scores. Assessment-as-Learning focuses particularly on assessment in its formative role, which is also the principal focus here.

4. Georgine Loacker, former Chair of the Assessment Council at Alverno, served as a consultant for the AACP Focus Group on Liberalization of the Professional Curriculum, created by the Commission to Implement Change in Pharmacy Education for the purpose of developing "outcome measures in designing curriculums and assessing student learning." Grants by the Fund for the Improvement of Post-Secondary Education (FIPSE) enabled pharmacy educators to apply ability-based methods to pharmacy education and to disseminate results.

   See American Association of Colleges of Pharmacy. Background Paper II: Entry-Level, Curricular Outcomes, Curricular Content and Educational Process [1990]. Commission to Implement Change in Pharmaceutical Education. Am J Pharm Educ 1993;57:377-85. Chalmers R, Grotpeter J, Hollenbeck R, et al. Ability-based outcome goals for the professional curriculum: a report of the Focus Group on Liberalization of the Professional Curriculum. Am J Pharm Educ 1992;56:304-9. Chalmers R, Grotpeter J, Hollenbeck G, Nickman N, Sommi R, Zlatic T. Changing to an outcome-based, assessment guided curriculum: a report of the Focus Group on Liberalization of the Professional Curriculum. Am J Pharm Educ 1994;58:108-15.

   Examples in pharmacy include: Purkerson D, Mason H, Chalmers R, Popovich G, Scott S. Evaluating pharmacy students' ability-based educational outcomes using an assessment center approach. Am J Pharm Educ 1996;60: 239-48. Purkerson D, Mason H, Chalmers R, Popovich G, Scott S. Expansion of ability-based education using an assessment center approach with pharmacists as assessors. Am J Pharm Educ 1997; 61:241-8. Vrahnos D, Dahdal W, Zlatic T, Maddux M. The peripheral brain: a tool to foster higher-order thinking in abilities-based courses. Am J Pharm Educ 1998;62:44-9. Vrahnos D, Maddux M. Introductory clinical clerkship during the first and second professional year: emphasis in clinical practice and writing. Am J Pharm Educ 1998;62:53-61. Perrier D, Winslade N, Pugsley J, Lavack L, Strand L. Designing a pharmaceutical care curriculum Am J Pharm Educ 1995; 59:113-24. Wallace C, Franson K. Incorporation of ability-based outcome education into pharmacotherapeutics using an expanded SOAP format. Am J Pharm Educ 1996;60:87-92. For an attempt to use the CAPE outcomes within experiential education, see Turner CJ, Altiere R, Clark L, Maffeo C, Valdez C. Competency-based introductory pharmacy practice experiential courses. Am J Pharm Educ 2005;69(2):article 21.

5. For an overview of ABE at the curriculum level, see Zlatic T. Abilities-based assessment within pharmacy education: Preparing students for practice of pharmaceutical care. In Wilkins NE, ed. Handbook for Pharmacy Educators: Contemporary Teaching Principles and Strategies. New York: Haworth Press 2000: 5-27. And see Maddux M. Institutionalizing assessment as learning within an ability-based program. In Wilkins NE, ed. Handbook for Pharmacy Educators: Contemporary Teaching Principles and Strategies, New York: Haworth Press 2000, 141-60. For a review of competency-based approaches in medical education, see Carraccio C, Wolfsthal SD, Englander R, Ferentz K, Martin C. Shifting paradigms: From Flexner to competencies. Acad Med 2002;77(5): 385-91.

6. Different definitions should not blind us to unanimity of purpose and design. For instance, IOM in its report, Health Professions Education, defines "competencies" very similarly to what we are in this chapter calling "abilities": "Competencies are defined here as the habitual and judicious use of communication, knowledge, technical skills, clinical reasoning, emotions, values, and reflections in daily practice" (pp. 3-4). Similarly, IOM uses the terms "competency-based" or "outcome-based" (OBE) education instead of ability-based education (pp. 89-90), but the goals and strategies are very similar. For some people, the term "OBE" has been politicized, sometimes indicating external bureaucratic control of the educational process, particularly in the public school system, whereas ability-based education emphasizes control by faculty and local administrators. And for some people, "ability" has a richer, more humanistic, and less technical connotation than does "competency," emphasizing the need to integrate general abilities into professional education. But what is important is not the terminology but the method of using carefully developed outcome statements to structure and assess learning.

7. Alverno College characterizes abilities as being integrated ("multiple components including skills, behaviors, knowledge, values, attitudes, motives or dispositions, and self-perceptions"), developmental ("pedagogical, cumulative levels that describe increasingly complex elements or processes"), and transferable ("they prepare students for many roles and settings"). Student assessment-as-learning at Alverno College. Milwaukee, WI: Alverno College Institute, 1994:9.

8. Epstein RM, Hundert EM. Defining and Assessing Professional Competence. JAMA 2002;287:226-7.

9. These outcomes/criteria were created at the St. Louis College of Pharmacy by committees headed by Jack Burke (thinking) and Brenda Gleason (self learning).

10. Zlatic TD, Nowak DM, Sylvester D. Integrating general and professional education through a study of herbal products: An intercollegiate collaboration. Am J Pharm Educ 2000;64:83-94.

11. See Bonwell C, Eison J. Active learning: creating excitement in the classroom. ASHE-ERIC Higher Education Report No. 1 Washington DC: The George Washington University, School of Education and Human Development, 1991. McKeachie W, Pintrich P, Lin Y, Smith D. Teaching and learning in the college classroom. Ann Arbor: University of Michigan, 1986.

12. Helpful is Stevens DD, Levi A. Introduction to rubrics: an assessment tool to save grading time, convey effective feedback, and promote student learning. Sterling, VA: Stylus Publishing, 2005.

13. Student assessment-as-learning at Alverno College. Milwaukee, WI: Alverno College Institute, 1994.

14. This example is taken from Electronic Student Portfolio (ESP), developed by Sheldon Holstad at the St. Louis College of Pharmacy. It is a Web-based portfolio system that employs an Assessment-as-Learning approach that places primary emphasis on improvement in student abilities.

Chapter 7: Writing to Learn in Pharmacy Education

> The relation between thought and word is a living process; thought is born through words. A word devoid of thought is a dead thing, and a thought unembodied in words remains a shadow.
>
> *L.S. Vygotsky*

How desirable or practical, in your opinion, is the following recommendation from the AACP Commission to Implement Change in Pharmaceutical Education?

> Most, if not all, [pharmacy] courses would require written assignments. Examinations should provide for written analyses of problems. Because written works usually require several revisions before excellence is achieved, the educational process must reflect this and students should be provided the opportunities to revise their papers based on constructive criticism from faculty and peers.[1]

Though both written and oral communication are recognized as increasingly important for practitioners who provide pharmaceutical care, many educators nonetheless have found such an emphasis on writing to be inordinate or impossibly ideal, particularly those educators who assume that the practice of writing mainly concerns itself with grammar, punctuation, and mechanics. Of course writing to communicate is an important ability outcome for most academic programs, but more central to the recommendation above is the realization that writing also can be a tool to discover, create, analyze, clarify, and evaluate ideas.

An intimate connection pertains between language and thought. It is naive to think that we, as adults, first have ideas and then find language to express them. What is labeled by the word "thinking" is in reality a complex, multidimensional set of mental processes, a number of which do occur without words. We can have ineffable experiences, and we can think spatially and imagistically or have flashes of insight in which, for instance, we can discover the DNA structure through a dream image of entwined serpents. But normally, when we analyze and deliberate discursively, words are the midwives of our ideas, if not their physical embodiment.[2] Language, then, not only has an expressive and a communicative aspect but also helps to generate ideas still being formed. This phenomenon may be even more apparent in writing. "We write," says C. Day Lewis, "not to be understood; we write in order to understand."

Human understanding often has a dialogic structure. In dialogue with others, we can broaden our perspectives and deepen our understanding as we learn from them what we did not know. But the process is not merely accretive. Imprisoned in ourselves as we are, we need interaction with others to understand not just what they think and know but what we ourselves know and believe. Unless challenged, we often will not recognize our beliefs and unquestioned assumptions. They exist as an invisible framework guiding our thinking. E. M. Forster's quip, "How do I know what I think until I see what I say?" rings true for those of us who have experienced the formulation of our opinions *during* discussion as we announce

> Most, if not all, [pharmacy] courses would require written assignments. Examinations should provide for written analyses of problems. Because written works usually require several revisions before excellence is achieved, the educational process must reflect this and students should be provided the opportunities to revise their papers based on constructive criticism from faculty and peers.
>
> *Commission to Implement Change in Pharmaceutical Education*

positions we never knew we had before. The encounter with another forces us to look inside ourselves and to take positions and/or to clarify our reasons for holding them.

Because of this, writing has tremendous implications and potential for curricular reform that strives for a student-centered pedagogy stressing active and life-long learning as students develop such abilities as critical thinking, communication, and problem solving within professional contexts. Such a cognitive/constructivist educational model necessitates significant innovation, as recognized by then AACP President Robert E. Smith in his 1999 inaugural address: "Maintaining a pharmaceutical content paradigm and trying harder to integrate the general education outcomes into our curricula will not be successful. We have to create a new curriculum that truly integrates professional education with the general education outcomes."[3]

Problem-based learning, case studies, simulations, active learning, early experiential activities, service learning, assessment as learning, and ability-based assessment are among the educational strategies colleges of pharmacy around the country are experimenting with in an effort to create this new curriculum. Not surprisingly, many of these strategies are likely to entail some component of writing in the preparation or presentation stages, for writing is a particularly powerful tool for learning. Many educators have found that if they want to learn a subject, the best method is to teach it and the next best method is to write an article about it. If the goal is for students to gain proficiency in problem solving, critical thinking, communication, and ethical decision making within professional contexts, writing deserves a more prominent role in the education of future practitioners. This chapter attempts to provide a rationale and some strategies for using writing as one means for helping students to develop the abilities they will need in their professional careers. Writing can be a stepping-stone toward the creation of a curricular paradigm that is content-rich and ability-centered.

Writing and General Ability Outcomes

Writing is a technology that conveys our ideas but, most important, also helps us formulate them. Of course, no magical transformations occur during the transcription of spoken words because simply writing things down does not enhance thinking. The act of putting pen to paper is not the essence of writing; rather, the transformative power of writing is in part connected to the different relationships that writing establishes with time and with the senses. Writing, when interiorized culturally and individually, can influence what we think and how we think.[4]

A brief reflection can support this. What are the possibilities of passing a therapeutics course if a student is not allowed to read, take notes, or in any way transcribe or record the lectures? How many people in pharmacy practice, students or professors, walk around with the contents of "DiPiro" or "Koda Kimble" in their heads? Obviously, writing is a tremendous aid to memory. Prior to the invention of writing, human knowledge was limited mostly to what could be retained in living human minds. In preliterate cultures people developed much more prodigious memories than most of us now, but not even they could memorize a therapeutics textbook, for obviously, without writing, the book (i.e., the body of knowledge) never could have been produced in the first place. Writing externalizes memory.

It is not merely the amount of knowledge that we are talking about here, but the complexity as well. Before writing, pharmacology, and all other "disciplines" consisted of observation captured in formulaic phrasing, proverbs, tales, and other conventional forms to serve as *aides-memoire*, such as, "Desperate diseases must have desperate cures"; "Bitter pills may have blessed effects"; "*Similia similibus curantur*" ("Like cures like"); "Eat leeks in oile and ramsines in May, And all the year after physicians may play"; "Don't step over the pennyroyal, dear"; "If you would live forever, you must wash milk from your liver"; "Cider on beer, never fear; beer upon cider, makes a bad rider." Writing enables the documented detailed observation, analytic thinking, and discursive practices that allow such oral tradition to develop into science. Historically, such characteristics of writing, and a *fortiori* of printing, have had such a tremendous impact on our thought and culture that even in this century of remarkable human achievements, it is not surprising that end-of-the-millennium pundits have identified the most influential discovery of the past thousand years to be a 16th century machine, the printing press.

> We write not to be understood;
> we write in order to understand.
>
> C. Day Lewis

Writing orients us differently toward our world. Spoken words are ephemeral, sounds constantly going out of existence as they are spoken. In writing, on the other hand, words and ideas appear to be "fixed," spatially available for detailed visual inspection. Unlike the auditor in a lecture, the reader can progress at one's own pace, stop to reflect, reread a passage, start over, or skip to the end. Moreover, with writing a person can place two or more texts side by side for comparison, can underline or circle text, write comments in a margin, entering into an imagined "conversation" with an author who may have been dead for many years. This externalization of knowledge, and a resulting distancing of the knower from the known, frees the mind from the onus of memory, making available additional psychic energy for more rigorous analysis.

"I hate writing because it makes you think." The student who uttered these words was on to something. Again, there are many types of writing and thinking, but discursive writing that is well done requires us to become engaged in more rigorous thinking than is usually necessary, or possible, in most ordinary conversations. The long pauses in the writing process as we stare at our computer screens, more than a silent search for the right word or grammatical nuance, are a groping for the right thought or the necessary evidence to support our claim. Fortunately, in speaking unaided by writing we normally are not required to announce a thesis, to organize our words around topics sentences, or to support our topic sentences with evidence and well-reasoned arguments. In some types of writing we are. Frequent writing (and reading) reinforces such thinking skills as generalization, division, and classification as we identify or formulate main points, subordinate supporting points, and order and arrange according to an emerging structure.

To write with authority, I need to be aware of and know how to find what others have said about my topic, to comprehend what they wrote, to paraphrase it, to analyze it, and to evaluate it. To be effective, I must provide detail and examples to support my claims, acknowledge when such evidence is partial or unavailable, understand the nature of evidence in my discipline, recognize the gaps in my thinking, probe my misconceptions, and modify my ideas in light of what I have discovered. Of course such processes could be incorporated into an oral presentation, but given how ingrained writing is in our scholarly enterprises, it is unlikely that such would occur without some preparation in writing.[5]

The temporal lag that writing grants between production and "publication"—the ability to pause during the writing process, to reflect, to search, and revise—distinguishes writing from speaking. The unscripted orator or conversationalist, pressured to "perform" before a live audience, is always constrained by ideas and memories currently in consciousness. In existential interactions, we do not have the opportunity to "revise" our statements or to freeze our audience while we seek additional thought or research. Everyone has experienced lying in bed at night remembering a verbal exchange during the day, and imagining the retort or the suggestion he or she should have made. Writing, with the lapses of time that exist between event and utterance, allows for that *mot juste*, that precise example or witty retort we wish we had thought of.

The "tax" for such temporal freedom is a concomitant requirement to be more focused in writing, to be hypersensitive regarding unity, organization, and clarity. Without changes in audible tone, gestures, and other contextual clues to clarify meanings, writing requires us to be precise, to anticipate rather than respond to audience confusion, and to give an architectonic shape to our ideas. Conversation is replete with diversions, free associations, and stream-of-consciousness wanderings, which is clear when we try to read transcriptions of conversations as in the infamous Watergate tapes, or on bad days, in our own lectures. Formal writing, on the other hand, downplays associative thought and directs us to stay focused and to be precise in thought and language as we weave our words with the words of others who have commented on the same topic. As I sit at my desk, fleshing out this paragraph, it may take me 20 minutes or more to organize and write what I could have said, though not as precisely, in 20 seconds. And it is not uncommon to spend 40–80 hours writing an article that might take 20 minutes to read. Of course it can take as much time to prepare a 20-minute speech, but it is unlikely in a contemporary Western, literate culture that during the preparation no writing or note-taking would be employed. Writing helps us to "keep" a thought, to integrate it with other thoughts, to give our thinking a structure, and to determine what our thoughts are. At the end of sophisticated writing projects, we know, perhaps for the first time, what we think, what our position is. If we have not to some degree modified our initial hypothesis, have not to some extent changed or enlarged our viewpoint, we might wonder if the effort was worthwhile.

It may be obvious that writing can help students achieve communication and thinking general ability outcomes, but it also can be an educational tool for developing other general abilities such as self and social awareness, ethical decision-making, valuing, and social interaction.

Separated from the give-and-take world of live dialogue, the writer and reader become more "distant" from their subject matter and their context. Composing alone, in the privacy of their own rooms, apart from an ongoing social interaction, writers are likely to be less emotionally and psychologically engaged, more able to focus on the idea itself and less on the context. Removed from face-to-face interpersonal dynamics, decontextualized from a specific time, place and occasion, the writer and reader are encouraged to be less polemical, more objective and analytic than they might be in a rhetorical debate. Writing can stimulate reflection and analysis.

Writing can also help us to recognize and combat a confining egocentricity. Writing paradoxically is more private, in that usually when writing we seclude ourselves from others and withdraw into our own consciousness, but also more public, for the results of our writing are not limited to an immediate time and precise place. In writing we expose ourselves and our thinking to all who might find the trace of our thoughts on the paper (or screen) in front of them. In light of these potentially distant and possibly not even yet born individuals, we must create both an audience and a context for our imagined dialogue. To do so we must move outside of our own thinking: to imagine their thoughts and feelings; to anticipate their goals, motivation, and prejudices; to play with multiple perspectives; to acknowledge our biases; to bring our assumptions to consciousness. In the absence of verbal and gestural responses from our audience that would cue us regarding their degree of understanding or agreement or interest or assent, we must create for ourselves anticipatory feedback. We must project the possible responses to our words and revise accordingly. Once we get our ideas "outside of ourselves" on the page, we are in a better position to dissociate them from ourselves, to treat them more objectively.

Writing To Learn

What I have written above can imply at least two misconceptions. First, writing is not inherently liberating or thought-provoking (just as philosophy does not always lead to wisdom nor theology to God). If not adequately prepared, students can respond even to meaningful assignments with "cognitively immature organizational structures" such as "and then" writing, which provides merely a chronological presentation of facts.[6] "All about" writing presents an encyclopedic overview without real purpose, and "data dump" writing randomly lists facts. And in fact, writing can discourage thinking. Some written assignments and tests, for instance, require students simply to repeat what was taught and memorized without comprehension, much less analysis or critique. The form and content of some writing can perpetuate stereotypes and stereotypical ways of thinking that can imprison rather than liberate, and of course written propaganda can intentionally deaden rather than encourage thought. Used, intentionally or unreflectively, as a social or ideological weapon, writing can be a form of oppression that privileges one race, gender, or social class and represses others. Excessive attention to mechanics and conventions during the writing process can stifle creativity and independent thinking.[7] Writing is a tool for exploration and clarification, but one must first learn how to use the tool and then must desire to use it for the purpose of truth-seeking.

Second, I have been speaking as if all writing were one process. Just as there are many types of thinking, there are many types of writing and many purposes for writing, many or most of which occur outside the academy. Academic writing itself incorporates many genres, including essays, critiques, summaries, lab reports, journals, reflection papers, patient education pamphlets, drug information papers, chart notes, Web page authoring, and a wide variety of writing-to-learn activities. Aside from genres, another way to categorize writing is based upon purpose. Two influential categories in the writing movement are "expressive writing" (informal writing that focuses on exploration of ideas, values, and relationships) and "communicative" or "transformational" writing (formal writing with an emphasis on conveying information to an audience).[8]

Traditionally, many writing-to-learn programs emphasize informal or "expressive writing," writing whose primary purpose is not to communicate but to "think out loud" on paper to discover new ideas or relationships between old and new ideas. Such expressive writing is not intended primarily for public consumption or judgment. Released from authoritarian external pressures and the fear of making mistakes, the expressive writer can risk exploration of ideas. Such writing forms as journals, diaries, brainstorming, and free-writes allow students to make connections between what they are learning and their own life world, their own mental constructs and values. In so doing, they begin to appropriate ownership of their knowledge and to recognize the temporal and conditional nature of knowledge production. Feminist critiques of science teaching and science writing, for instance, have applauded expressive, nontraditional writing as an antidote to the sexist and ethnocentric values and paradigms pervasive in the discipline.[9]

Some writing-to-learn techniques are brief and informal, involving both expressive writing and "short writes" geared toward learning content or skill.[10] The minute (or five-minute) essay is an active learning strategy to engage students in the learning process. At the beginning of class the technique is used to focus students on the topic by having them summarize a reading assignment or the previous lecture, or by writing an answer to a question raised when class begins. To recapture student attention during a lecture, the instructor can ask students to write questions or comments about what is not clear, to solve a problem, or to exchange and critique notes taken during class. At the end of class, the writing strategy can be used to have students identify the main points of the lecture, to find unresolved issues, to connect what was learned to previous classes or to personal experiences or to current events. Such short writes can be kept in student learning journals or can be transcribed onto 3-by-5 note cards that the instructor can pick up and assess.

Another writing strategy is for students to keep a diary or log in which they record observations and insights, conduct brainstorming, and establish connections between what they are now learning and their previous knowledge and experiences. A variation is the double-entry journal in which students record on one column of a page a summary of what they have read or experienced and then on a second parallel column write the questions, connections, and responses to what they have read and seen. Asking students to write test questions can stimulate them to find patterns in what they are learning and can encourage metacognition. Directed reading assignments pose a series of questions that students must answer in writing as they read an article or chapter. These questions can steer students to find key points, require students to show that they have comprehended what they read, and possibly direct students to respond to the text either by analyzing or evaluating. Comprehension and analysis are promoted by a one-sentence summary in which students digest a reading selection into one sentence, perhaps using a predetermined format consisting of the questions of Who? Does what? To whom/what? When? Where? How?

and Why? The primary motivation behind these strategies is not to improve students' writing abilities but to develop thinking skills and to master content.

In many of these cases the writing requires a kind of "translation" of course content. Students must internalize the subject matter, integrate it with previous conceptions and misconceptions, relate it to one's everyday experiences, and explain it in terms of analogies to persons unfamiliar with the topic. For instance, physics students who must explain the laws of acceleration to their significant others, using a pop fly in baseball as an example, must extend their knowledge beyond rote memorization of some definitions or formulaic calculations.[11] When they have finished writing, the knowledge is not simply layered in their brains as another stratum of data that probably soon will be eroded; rather, it has been "absorbed" into their thought processes, integrated with their past learning. It is not uncommon for college graduates after a number of years to forget even taking some college courses but to remember with vivid detail writing assignments they completed 20–30 years earlier.

Expanding the Concept of Writing to Learn

Although writing can be a means for students to translate science into terms and concepts within their everyday experiences, to adapt scientific concepts to their own models of understandings and expectations, and to develop personal ownership of ideas, it is also important to widen and adapt the students' paradigms and thinking processes to those within science. Writing within traditional scientific genres may help to accomplish that. Each discipline has its own models, with the differences being more substantive than mere conventions or formatting. Learning to write in a discipline is a form of enculturation in which students learn the patterns of thinking, habitual models of organization, and values of that discipline.

> If you cannot—in the long run—tell everyone what you have been doing, your doing has been worthless.
>
> *Erwin Schrödinger*

Unfortunately, a too narrow understanding of writing to learn may have helped to precipitate controversies regarding writing to learn in the sciences. The need for students, particularly in the early years of education, to create and appropriate for themselves intellectual and emotional bridges to science and the desire to release women and minorities from a tyranny of thought associated with masculine, Western experiences, are both strong arguments for expressive writing as a teaching tool. However, writing to learn is not limited to short, self-directed exploratory writing.

The debates over writing to learn approaches are complicated by shifting terminology.[12] First, pigeonholing writing into such categories as poetic, expressive, transactional, and mechanical, while obviously useful for analytic and pedagogical purposes, can oversimplify the complexity of writing and obscure the overlapping of categories in any one piece of writing. Too often terms slide into binary classifications: expressive writing or communicative/ transactional/expository writing; articulation or communication; informal or formal writing; /metacognitive/ heuristic/epistemic writing or reportorial writing; knowledge-telling modes or knowledge transforming modes. Writing to learn pedagogy, of course, by definition, favors those approaches that are constructivist, heuristic and metacognitive, those that make meaning rather than merely convey it. But that does not mean that all exploratory writing is private and informal or that all formal writing is only transactional. Unfortunately, in the above dichotomies, communication sometimes is relegated to "mere" status. That is, in this model "communicative" writing is too quickly associated only with procedures for assessing students, and students "communicate" to the instructor what they have been told and memorized.

But this is an impoverished sense of what communication is: telling something to someone who already knows it for the purpose of judging whether or not the teller really knows it as well. Communication in writing normally is a much richer and more complex activity that entails identifying a purpose for communication and an audience to communicate with; analyzing that audience and trying on a different point of view; finding, selecting and arranging, and synthesizing ideas and arguments that will be convincing to that audience; identifying, critiquing, and employing interpretive frameworks; identifying one's own assumptions and prejudices; solving problems; and revising in light of new insights and discoveries. Transactional writing can be and often is information-centered, with the purpose of clearly conveying facts, not analyzing or challenging them. This is not a trivial ability, for as quantum physicist Erwin Schrödinger stated, "If you cannot—in the long run—tell everyone what you have been doing, your doing has been worthless."[13] But writing for an audience also can be problem-based, research-oriented, analytical, or argumentative, allowing the writer to undertake investigations which probably would not be attempted, or perhaps even be possible, without the writing project. If this is how communication is defined, it is more obvious that communicative writing is a sophisticated method for writing to learn. It is concerned not merely with knowledge transmission but with knowledge production. As John Updike says, "Writing and rewriting are a constant search for what one is saying."

There are more compelling arguments for the use of formal writing in the sciences. The connection of writing to science extends much deeper than writing's use as a pedagogical tool. In the introduction to Halliday and Martin's *Writing Science: Literacy and Discursive Power*, Alan Luke alludes to historical, anthropological evidence that "writing is the enabling technology for 'doing' modern science." Although it might be more precise to state that print, more than just writing, was the fuel which fired the scientific revolution,[14] worth pursuing is Luke's claim that the technicality and abstraction of modern science are not thinkable in the language of everyday life, and thus it is "naive pedagogy" to think that effective science education can totally escape the language or jargon of science.[15]

Once again, as several thinkers such as Marshall McLuhan, Walter Ong, and Jack Goody have shown, language not merely represents reality but can help to structure it; and likewise, the modes by which language is expressed (orality, writing, print, electronic technology) are not neutral, passive agents or inert "media" between the speaker/writer and listener/reader or between the knower and the known. Writing, for instance, is an internal technology that enables, and discourages, ways of thinking and ways of interacting with others. Along these lines, Halliday and Martin argue that the language of science does not simply mirror nature more rigorously or in closer detail than does ordinary language. Its lexogrammatical features, its vocabulary and grammar, actually facilitate the construction of categories that may be literally "unthinkable" in everyday language. "The language of science is, by its nature, language in which theories are constructed. Its special features are exactly those that make theoretical discourse possible."[16] In short, substantive, systematic changes in lexicon grammar can influence changes in conceptualization. This is not to say that scientific language is the perfect, immutable symbol system in which language and reality correspond precisely, for scientific language and patterns of organization, like all language and patterns of organization, are social/ideological processes that select, valorize, and thematize. They expand and reveal at the same time they limit and distort. Students must recognize that science and the language of science are value-laden, socially constructed, and subject to continual evolution.[17] If students are to learn not just facts but the power to establish facts, learning to write within disciplinary genres and formats can be an enabling step. They must first understand the language regardless if they seek to perpetuate or change it.

Thus "writing to learn" can refer to short, writer-centered, mostly ungraded writing assignments that encourage students to explore a subject and their reactions to it, without much attention to conventions or audience. But it is a mistake to think that audience-directed and more disciplined writing assignments do not encourage students to learn from their writing. Both types of writing have advantages, and within a well-planned curriculum, expressive writing can be used to "scaffold" to more formal assignment within traditional scientific disciplines, such as experiment, explanation, report, biography, and exposition.[18] In that way students can understand facts and ideas in terms of their existing conceptual frameworks, gradually adapting their patterns of language and thinking to frameworks of their disciplines. Through increasingly sophisticated writing projects, they will see better how knowledge in their disciplines is created, assessed, and modified. They are more likely to become educated rather than trained.

And in fact, writing assignments can be constructed to address all the thinking levels listed in Bloom's taxonomy. At the lowest level, writing assignments can be used to evaluate whether or not students have retained information. Moving up, many of the writing assignments described above are successful in helping students comprehend subject matter because they require students to paraphrase for a "lay" audience such disciplinary concepts as bioavailability, metabolism, photosynthesis, resonance, or capitation. Students cannot simply repeat terms and explanations they do not understand, as they might on a written exam in which recall rather than comprehension is being tested. Other writing assignments require students to apply their knowledge, such as writing background and other explanatory material to put into perspective chemistry-related articles appearing in newspapers, or applying the theory of utilitarianism to an ethical dilemma regarding a conflict between the principle of confidentiality and concern for the public good. As we have seen, writing promotes analysis. If students were not required to write an analysis/discussion section of a lab report or technical paper, it is questionable whether they would ever understand as clearly and precisely what occurred during the experiment. Some writing assignments challenge students to synthesize, as in physiology when students are asked to invent and explain a pheromone. In evaluative essays, students use compelling evidence to make insightful judgments regarding the value, correctness, or desirability of an idea or action, such as the practice of third-party payments, legalization of pharmacist prescribing, the efficacy and safety of complimentary and alternative medicines, roles for pharmacy technicians, or issues in mail and Internet dispensing.

The literature is replete with claims of the efficacy of using writing to develop disciplinary thinking.[19] Students in math classes work in learning groups to express in writing their conceptual understanding of calculus, with the result that both their cognitive abilities and their attitudes toward learning improve.[20] A study of writing projects in second semester chemistry determined that "the completion of frequent critical-thinking writing assignments is a more effective way to learn chemical concepts than traditional drill-type exercises,"[21] and similar conclusions are reached regarding the efficacy of writing to learn in organic chemistry.[22] In a statistics class, students outperformed a control group when they wrote jargon-free press releases regarding the statistical problems they were investigating.[23] Students in biology who had frequent writing assignments integrated into their course were better able to understand biology and to evaluate data, with 60% of those students making "significantly higher grades in ... subsequent classes than did comparable students who did not take the course."[24] Within nursing, writing is used as a method to develop critical thinking to enable practitioners to "select appropriate information and defend its integration into patient care."[25] And in pharmacy, students enrolled in a section of verbal communication that employed "language-for-learning" techniques showed improvement in writing skills, ability to formulate ideas, and identifying appropriate target audiences, whereas students in a control section did not.[26]

Pharmacy Applications

Applications to pharmacy education are unlimited. Every class, regardless of size or content, can employ writing-to-learn techniques that promote active learning, such as short writes, minute essays, and directed readings. Longer assignments are also excellent teaching tools in every area of pharmacy. Patient information pamphlets (and now videos with written scripts) require students to understand complicated information so that they can explain it in lay terms. With the growth of online pharmacies, a valuable writing assignment is to have students provide clear and accurate electronic responses to simulated patient queries provided over the Internet. Herbal products and alternative therapies provide opportunities for integrating general and professional abilities through writing. The problem patients have with herbal medicines is not insufficient information but an overabundance of it, much of it unsubstantiated or patently wrong. A writing assignment that requires students first to analyze herbal advertising and scientific data relating to herbal medicines and then to write monographs for patient education is an exercise in communication as well as in analysis and evaluation, preparing students to counsel and educate patients.[27] Clearly, accurately, and completely documenting drug therapy assessment and recommendations in the medical records can develop pharmacist accountability and professional credibility in a collaborative primary care practice. Teaching pharmacy students to write chart notes can be a useful way to evaluate their professional abilities to assess and recommend drug therapies.[28]

Journals exploit the expressive function of writing. For instance, within pharmacy education and elsewhere, service learning has been heralded as an excellent opportunity for students to explore their assumptions, values, prejudices, social/civic responsibilities, and the meaning of their professional commitment to pharmaceutical care.[29] By performing volunteer work with underserved populations and individuals in need, students accumulate experiences that encourage intellectual, emotional, and professional growth. Once again, writing can be the catalyst for insightful reflection. Often in service learning, students make weekly entries in a journal to distill their volunteer experiences and reach insightful conclusions. Usually instructors who read the journals are less concerned about grammar and structure or about communicating objectively and convincingly with a wide audience. The primary purpose is to discover what students think and feel and believe. This does not mean, of course, that journal writing is "ungradable" fluff, for specific criteria for the entries can be established. For instance, the writer should: objectively observe and describe what took place; explain his or her subjective responses to what happened; analyze the volunteering experiences in order to find patterns, explanations, and causes; evaluate both what took place and one's responses to what happened; and devise plans for enhanced performance at the next volunteer opportunity. Such criteria have prospective as well as retrospective benefits, for knowing that they will need to fulfill the criteria in their next journal entries, students at their sites become more observant regarding events and environment, more alert and inquisitive, more attentive to what can be changed to improve their performance and the well-being of their patients/clients. Because of the need to reflect in writing upon their experiences, the students are "predisposed" to learning when they enter their sites. The journal entry then provides the opportunity to sift through their sensory experiences, their emotional responses, and their thoughts in order to better understand themselves, those they work with, and the nature of their profession. If pharmaceutical care requires caring for as well as caring about patients, such expressive writing should be incorporated into a number of courses throughout the curriculum.[30]

Disease monographs for health-care collaborators provide opportunities for students to learn and remember content as they experiment with adapting communication to different audiences. Drug information papers teach students content, critical analysis, and scientific thinking. Argumentative essays extend the knowledge and thinking skills of students as they explore the background and find evidence to support positions on such topics as the nature of pharmaceutical care, the appropriate uses of Ritalin, ethical issues in pharmacy practice, or compensation for cognitive services. Analytic memos are problem-solving simulations in which students write concise plans to address, for instance, a problem arising in a pharmacy or nursing home. Or students can write essays to propose strategies to increase patient compliance regarding specific drugs and disease states. Of course, having students write both cases and solutions to cases allows them to practice problem-solving strategies. Problem solving can also be encouraged by having students write business plans. Requiring students to keep journals during rotations can help them and their preceptors to monitor cognitive and attitudinal development. In pharmacy and other professions, it is important to instruct students on "writing" within an electronic environment using new conventions, formats, and genres associated with e-mail, bulletin boards, Web page production, and online presentations.

In these writing assignments, learning is enhanced if students rewrite. Writing is recursive. It instantiates the hermeneutical circle: How can we know the whole until we understand the parts, but how can we understand the parts until we know the whole? Revision is one strategy. Make an attempt to create a structure based upon what is known, "re-see" what is known in light of that structure, modify the structure in light of what has been re-seen, and repeat the process. As opposed to editing, which is oriented more toward conventions, revision is the process of rethinking the writing assignment. Assessment can be a catalyst for such rethinking. If students are given clear criteria at the time the assignment is given, they can self-assess their work before they turn it in. For more objective feedback, peers can assess according to the same criteria, with an advantage being that the peers come to a better understanding of what constitutes successful performance through specific examples. In marking papers, instructors can point out problems, challenge ideas, suggest new lines of thinking; however, if the student is not required to rewrite the essay, it is unlikely that he or she will benefit much from such comments, regardless of how perceptive and detailed they are. It is in the revision that the student must wrestle with the instructor's comments, modify frameworks, extend thinking, and come to a more accurate and complete understanding. Formative assessment provides the dialogue that encourages the student to discover what he or she is saying.

Developing Attitudes and Values through Writing

Persuasive essays in particular are effective in helping students develop knowledge and skills as well as attitudes and values. Because in a persuasive essay the audience by definition is someone who disagrees with you, the writer, you cannot rely solely on sound arguments backed up by reasons that are supported by sufficient and credible evidence to convince readers of your position. The persuasion process is as much psychological as logical, which is intuitive to any teenager who praises his father's golf game before asking for the keys to the car. The readers know that you disagree with them and therefore are defensive from the beginning. To be effective you must gain the respect of the readers, which you do by showing respect and exhibiting empathy. Before you can demonstrate the reasonableness and desirability of your position, you must establish rapport with the audience, building bridges as you find common ground, acknowledge their merits, and demonstrate your own good will, fairness, and competency. As a persuasive writer you must take the time to formulate and clarify your own position and understand what your audience believes, why they believe it, and why they believe you are wrong. As a persuasive writer, you must identify why your audience disagrees with you and be able to state their position as they would state it. Then you must tailor your arguments to their reasons, values, and concerns. Often during this process, the persuasion writer discovers that the issues are more complex than he or she first believed, and the audience is not as stupid or evil as perhaps first believed. Through the process of writing, the persuasive writer often modifies his or her own original position and becomes more open to compromise. In short, persuasive writing is an exercise in empathy. It requires us to escape the prison of egocentricity and try to take the perspective of other persons, to be concerned about finding out what people believe and why they believe it, rather than simply trying to enforce our own beliefs and values upon others.

Persuasion is difficult to write, and few students excel in their first versions. Even after being given criteria for effective persuasion, they often give only token attention to the audience, offering formulaic concessions to one or two minor points of the audience and then proceeding to their own agendas, ignoring the audience or even alienating them. Because they are unable to put themselves in the place of their audience, they do not recognize that the language they use is insensitive or offensive. For these reasons, persuasive writing often requires one or more revisions, based upon feedback. Peer assessment is an especially helpful tool, particularly when peers are asked to assume the role of the intended audience and to provide feedback about the tactics and arguments of the writer. And as is normally the case with peer assessment, the peer assessor benefits from the process, having a better understanding of the criteria and how to improve his or her own performance (see the end of the chapter for an example of peer assessment for persuasion).

Ideally the process results in a better writer and a better clinical practitioner. Patients who are in pain, afraid, or tired, who don't know how they can afford medical treatment, who come from other countries, or who speak foreign languages may perform many aggravating and incomprehensible actions. Students who have been successful in persuasion writing have a better appreciation for the need to see multiple viewpoints on any topic, less disdain for those who think differently then they do, and greater willingness to postpone judgment of others until they have taken the time to understand what they believe and why they are behaving they way they are. Topics such as use of complementary medicines or refusal of pharmacists to fill emergency contraception scripts can provoke many sometimes heated arguments. Asking students to write persuasively on the opposite side of what they believe on such issues can lead to better understanding. You cannot force anyone to be empathic, but you can put students in situations that tend to evoke empathic responses, in physical or mental spaces that require them to step outside themselves.

Conclusions

Thus "writing" in professional education does not refer to one activity or practice. A variety of writing activities can be adopted to achieve a variety of educational outcomes for students at varying points in their cognitive and affective development. Instructors can create writing assignments to encourage students to investigate and to appropriate content, to demonstrate comprehension, to develop analytical skills, to explore one's self and values, to interrelate disparate ideas, to synthesize, to develop disciplinary thinking, to understand one's audience, to argue using clear and compelling arguments, to perform professional abilities such as recommend drug therapies, educate and counsel patients, or collaborate with other health care professionals.

Though the dawning of an information age will put new demands on the communication abilities of pharmacists, it is a mistake to base the commitment to writing in pharmacy education solely upon the quantity and types of writing that are performed in professional practice. Of course students should learn to write clearly and effectively in the genres and formats they will be required to use as practitioners, but the primary purpose for incorporating writing throughout the curriculum is to educate, rather than merely train, professionals who provide pharmaceutical care. Such professionals will understand how knowledge is constructed, be self-aware and oriented toward others, be problem solvers who can find, understand, analyze, synthesize, evaluate, and communicate information. Writing as a way of learning is an example of how the integration of general and professional ability outcomes can produce professionals who can frame and solve problems.

Impracticalities of course abound in trying to incorporate significant writing into most pharmacy courses: class sizes, available time of both instructors and students, lack of instructor ability and/or comfort and/or desire in designing and assessing writing assignments. Some solutions exist. Faculty development programs can demonstrate the efficacy of writing as a teaching tool, teach the use of rubrics in assessing writing, and provide strategies for assessment as learning. Writing centers at most universities can provide ideas for creating and assessing writing assignments and support the instructor with direct assistance to students. Curriculum committees can propose across-the-curriculum plans for teaching and assessing writing as well as required writing emphasis courses in which students frequently practice writing and rewriting in order to learn a subject matter.[31]

However, such efforts alone probably will not be sufficient, for "curricular reform" extends beyond tacking writing onto existing courses that continue to constitute a content-centered curriculum. The addition of meaningful writing assignments into a curriculum can assist in a reconceptualization of what the purpose of education is within a pharmacy program. Using a cognitive/constructivist educational model, faculty can devise curricula and courses that integrate general and professional abilities to enable students to learn not just facts but the power to establish facts, to know the solutions for existing problems and achieve the ability to solve problems that have not yet presented themselves. Writing, a communication ability useful for any professional, is also a highly effective teaching tool to educate practitioners in ways that will help them develop the abilities to provide pharmaceutical care.

Some Tips and Tools for Writing to Learn

For those faculty who acknowledge the benefits of incorporating writing into professional courses, two primary deterrents to doing so are the amount of time it takes to assess assignments and the instructor's sense of inadequacy in assessing writing.

To address the latter first, one need not have a degree in English or Composition Studies to assess written work within one's own discipline. Although common student errors such as "misplaced modifiers, comma splices, and faulty parallelism" may be more unintelligible to the instructor than quantum theory, without such a specialized vocabulary the instructor can still evaluate whether or not the writing is clear, whether or not the logic is sound, whether enough evidence is provided to back up the claims made, whether the student achieves the outcomes for which the assignment was constructed. One's insecurities about one's own writing ability should not deprive students of opportunities to enhance their thinking and communication through writing.

Unfortunately, creating and assessing writing assignments do require a significant amount of time. And once class sizes exceed 25–30 students, even competent instructors who are enthusiastic about writing to learn may back off. Nonetheless, there are some strategies that can make some writing assignments manageable in classes of more than 100 or even 200 students. Here are some tips and tools for implementing writing to learn.

Grading Templates

A way to save time in grading while still providing detailed feedback is to use a template. On a handout specify the criteria you expect for the assignment, and on a separate sheet detail the mistakes that students are likely to make apropos each criterion. Distribute a copy of the criteria to each student when the assignment is made so they can

Some Strategies for Assessing Writing Assignments in Large Classes

- Don't grade written work.
  Sample student responses to assess what needs to be done in the classroom to improve student learning.
  Give group feedback regarding commonly made errors.
  Require revision of students whose work does not meet assignment outcomes.

- Grade only for selected criteria.
  Identify specific criteria for writing assignments and grade the writing project only on those criteria. Grammar/mechanics for example need not be a criterion if it is not relevant to the assignment.

- Grade selectively.
  Assign multiple writing tasks over the semester. Grade some assignments but not others, without announcing which will be graded and which will not.
  Grade 5 (or 10, 15) students randomly from each assignment. Ensure over the course of the semester that each student is assessed twice or more.
  Have students keep a portfolio of writing assignments. Collect two-three times a semester. Tell students to mark their 3 best entries. Grade those, plus 3 others selected randomly.

- Use holistic grading.
  Mark written work as either acceptable (T) or unacceptable (-); a (+) could be assigned for superior work. Give total credit or no credit. Allow students who have no credit to revise and re-submit.

- Create grading templates. (See below)
  Determine in advance the most common problems students will have with a writing assignment, and create a form or template that contains lengthy feedback on how to correct each problem. Duplicate the sheet and return to each individual student, calling attention to the template items that could help the student to improve.

- Require peer and self-assessment. (See below.)
  Create assessment sheets with clear criteria. When writing projects are given, distribute the assessment sheets. Have students assess their own and one other person's essays and then revise their own essays.

- Assign group projects.
  Assign writing projects in which students collaborate in teams of four, thus reducing by three-quarters the amount of written work needed to be graded.

- Refer students to the Writing Center.
  Writing Center staff can help identify and correct writing problems.

- Use Graders/Teaching Assistants.
  Train teaching assistants to grade using holistic scoring methods.

consult it as they are writing their essays. Then, while grading a student's work, write on the essay the number that corresponds to the error made by the student, or, alternatively, check the pertinent comments on the template, underlining or highlighting key points as needed. (Praise or encouraging words also can be put on the template, although sometimes it is more meaningful if such short comments are written directly on the essay).

The template remarks can be as detailed or general as you would like them. You can include explanations, examples, references for further help, even mini-lectures. For those who move around easily in electronic environments, the templates can be digitized, enabling feedback that contains sound and images and links to Web materials. The template comments can explain content issues, writing issues, or both. Students actually can be given more complete feedback this way than by hand-marking the essays. Of course, the instructor can mark comments on the essay when necessary.

It takes time to construct the template the first time it is used, but it is easily updated and capable of being modified to fit other assignments or classes. After you give the assignment, you can continually update the template to address common errors you did not at first think of.

Here are some sample comments that might be added to a grading template.

Grading Template

1. **One clear, central idea should be the basis for the organization of your essay.**
    1.1 An expository essay should have a thesis, a one-sentence summary of the main point of the essay. (See The Practical Writer, p. 34, for an explanation; see the Web site www.longy.writngcntr/lab).
    1.2 A thesis should be unified, making only one point. One way to correct problems with unity is to turn compound sentences into complex sentences. Example: Not unified—The economy is in terrible trouble, and most high school graduates can no longer afford to attend college. Unified—Because of the terrible economy, most high school graduates have great difficulty attending college.
    1.3 A thesis should be complete. It should include in it a summary of everything in the essay. Some issues in your essay are not reflected in the thesis.
    1.4 A thesis should be clear. Use precise words. Avoid general terms.
    1.5 A thesis should be limited. That is, you must not try to say too much in a short space. For a 500-word essay, your topic is too broad; you will not be able to say anything very meaningful about it. Narrow it down. Example: Too broad — College students today… Limited — Fourth year students at Smart College…
    1.6 Normally the thesis appears at the end of the introductory paragraph. It can be placed elsewhere, but if you do not have a specific reason for placing it elsewhere, put it at the end of the first paragraph.
    1.7 A thesis should be interesting and meaningful. Your thesis doesn't say much that most people don't already know. Try brainstorming about the issue. What is controversial about it? What would people want to know and why?

2. **You need to tailor your essay to your audience.**
   2.1   Who is your audience? What do they already know about your topic? Why do they want to know what you are telling them? It is not clear from your essay that you have given these questions enough thought.
   2.2   The tone you use in the essay alienates your audience. They will not be persuaded to accept your ideas if you ridicule their current position. Concede some issues. Try to state the position of your audience as they would state it. (See *Writing for Real Audiences*, p. 122, for an explanation.)
   2.3   The language you use is not appropriate for the audience for which you are writing. Do not use slang and colloquial terms here. (See the explanation at *www.tone.sampleexercise* and complete the exercises at the end of the lesson.)
   2.4   Your language is too technical for a lay audience…

3. **You do not clearly and completely critique the limitations of this article from the medical literature.**
   3.1   You do not comment about the number of patients in this study. Normally, … What criticisms can you make about the use of statistics in this article? For instance …

4. **You should take patient specific data more into consideration in selection of drug therapy.**
   4.1   You are correct in thinking that … but …

5. **Click here for to review the uses of primary, secondary, and tertiary literature.** [for digitized feedback]

6. **Look at how these three students employed secondary literature, and determine which of the three was most effective.** [Insert passages]. **How can your use of the secondary literature be improved?**

7. **It is important to follow the American Medical Association style sheet.**
   7.1   You do not cite sources properly. See the examples at *www.samplenote.assn1*.

Peer-Assessment: General Writing Skills

1. The writer had a clear, unified, and limited claim (thesis) that guided the essay.
   ___ yes   ___ to some degree   ___ no
   What is it?
   How can it be improved?

2. The writer used convincing, clearly stated reasons to support his or her claim.
   ___ yes   ___ to some degree   ___ no
   What are they?
   How can they be improved?

3. The writer provided sufficient evidence and logical explanations to support his or her reasons.
   ___ yes   ___ to some degree   ___ no
   What are the reasons?
   What can be improved?

4. The writer negotiated and/or refuted other perspectives on this issue.
   ___ yes   ___ to some degree   ___ no
   Where in the essay?
   How can it be improved?

5. The writer wrote paragraphs that are organized in a logical order and have clear topic sentences that are directly related to the thesis.
   ___ yes   ___ to some degree   ___ no
   What can be done better?

6. The writer developed the paragraphs and used sufficient specific details and examples.
   ___ yes   ___ to some degree   ___ no
   What can be done better?

7. The writer revised to clearly relate the parts of the essay to one another (coherence).
   ___ yes   ___ to some degree   ___ no
   What can be done better?

8. The writer revised to eliminate inaccurate or unclear statements.
   ___ yes   ___ to some degree   ___ no
   What can be done better?

9. The writer revised the essay to make it clear and fluid and eliminated choppy sentences and wordiness.
   ___ yes   ___ to some degree   ___ no
   What can be done better?

10. The writer edited to remove all grammatical, mechanical, and spelling errors.
    ___ yes   ___ to some degree   ___ no
    What can be done better?

Summary Self/Peer Assessment Form for Grading

I. In each category, check the <u>one</u> statement which <u>best</u> describes this essay:

1. <u>Main Idea</u>
   - a___ Very clearly stated, sophisticated idea that can be adequately covered in the space available
   - b___ Sophisticated idea but not always clear or sufficiently limited
   - c___ Clearly stated, meaningful, and limited basic idea
   - d___ Basic idea, not always clear or sufficiently limited; or insignificant idea covered adequately; not a meaningful topic
   - e___ Idea is unclear, too broad, and/or not significant

2. <u>Organization</u>
   - a___ Masterfully structured with effective transitions, clear topic sentences
   - b___ Clearly structured with effective transitions and topic sentences
   - c___ The reader at times must infer structure or supporting points
   - d___ Structure and/or relevance of material is not always clear or cannot be inferred
   - e___ Essay does not follow a clear plan, contains irrelevant information, confuses the reader

3. <u>Development</u>
   - a___ Convincing, logical arguments and adequate, specific evidence demonstrate the validity of the main point
   - b___ Sophisticated, logical arguments and concrete evidence are effectively used, but sometimes additional rigor and\or completeness is needed
   - c___ Basic arguments and evidence support the main idea, but either they may be somewhat incomplete, illogical, or based upon questionable assumptions. Lacks examples and details.
   - d___ Errors in logic or inadequate evidence and lack of examples lead the reader to question the conclusions
   - e___ Faulty or nonexistent arguments and evidence undermine the conclusions

4. <u>Insight</u>
   - a___ The essay presents an insightful viewpoint or perspective with illuminating examples and compelling arguments
   - b___ The writer clearly has something insightful to say but doesn't always have complete control over its formulation and/or presentation
   - c___ The writer presents useful, basic information and occasionally expresses insights that challenge the reader
   - d___ Basic information is presented but the reader does not learn much that is new
   - e___ The essay should not have been written because it expresses mostly obvious information that the reader already knows

5. <u>Conventions and Style</u>
   - a___ The essay demonstrates flawless grammar and mechanics; appropriate use of words; conscious selection of a tone that engages the reader
   - b___ Some minor but no major errors in grammar or mechanics; word choice mostly appropriate; the tone mostly engages the reader
   - c___ One major error in grammar or mechanics that does not interfere with clarity; words used are basic but clear and specific; tone does not alienate the reader
   - d___ One or more major errors in grammar/mechanics that cause confusion, or several major and minor errors; frequent spelling mistakes; word choice not always appropriate; inattention to tone
   - e___ Serious or multiple errors make reading difficult; words often are used inappropriately; tone alienates the reader

6. <u>Assignment Requirements</u>
   - a___ The essay fulfills the assignment's outcomes in an exemplary fashion; all requirements are met, including appropriate topic choice, length, procedures, timeliness
   - b___ The essay accomplishes the outcomes of the essay and follows all directions
   - c___ The essay meets the assignment outcomes, but does not comply completely with all directions regarding format, length, timeliness, as stipulated in the directions
   - d___ The essay, even if well-written, does not completely meet the assignment outcomes or consistently ignores directions
   - e___ The essay does not meet the outcomes for the assignment or does not meet clearly defined expectations stated in the directions

II. Use the grading scale below as a guideline to calculate the grade:

__A __A- __B+ __B __B- __C+ __C __C- __D+ __D __D- __F

- A = "A" line on all 6 items
- B+ = "A" line on all except "B" line in one or two on #1-4
- B- = "B" line on all except "C" line in one of #1-4
- C = mostly line "C"
- D+ = mostly lines "D" with some lines "C"
- D- = nothing higher than lines "D"

- A- = "A" line on #1-4 & "B" line in #5-6
- B = "B" line on all
- C+ = mostly "C" line with one or two "B" lines on #1-4
- C- = mostly lines "C" with one or two lines "D" on #5-6
- D = mostly lines "D"
- F = line "E" on any

Drug Information Paper: Assessment Form

Performance Criteria	Assess-ment Score	Evidence/Feedback
Evaluates biomedical literature.		
Uses pertinent primary sources (2 pts)		
Uses pertinent secondary sources (1 pt)		
Uses pertinent tertiary sources (2 pts)		

Summarizes methods, includes: (4 pts)
     a. study design
     b. variables
     c. outcome measures
     d. statistical method		

Summarizes results, includes: (4 pts)
     o outcome measures
     o tables, figures as necessary
     o clinical versus statistical significance		

Identifies strengths (2 pts)		
Identifies limitations (2 pts)		
Answers question posed in introduction (4 pts)		
Supports body of response (2 pts)		
Includes statement regarding strength of data or need for additional data (1 pt)		
States conclusions in appropriate length (5-10 lines) (1 pt)		
Communicates drug-related information to peers, patients, and other health care providers.		
Includes correct clinical case/question in introduction (2 pts)		
States introduction in appropriate length (5-10 lines) (2 pt)		
Writes an introduction that pertains to the question (3 pts)		
Uses effective transitions and clear topic sentences (3 pts)		
Cites specific evidence to support the question (4 pts)		
Presents an insightful viewpoint with examples (3 pts)		
Uses correct grammar (3 pts)		
Uses correct spelling (3 pts)		
Cites references appropriately according to guidelines for biomedical journals (2 pts)		

Peer Assessment: Persuasion Essay
Criteria-referenced, evidence-based feedback

1. How knowledgeable does the writer appear to be on this topic?
   ___ "expert" ___ well-informed ___ credible ___ neutral ___ questionable

   The writer shows he/she is knowledgeable by . . .
   The writer's knowledgeability is questionable when . . .
   The writer could improve in this area by . . .

2. How fair is the writer?
   ___ extremely fair ___ fair ___ mostly fair ___ sometimes not fair ___ "too fair"

   The writer demonstrates fairness when . . .
   The writer does not demonstrate fairness when . . .
   The writer could improve fairness by . . .

3. For this essay, who do you think is the intended audience; what beliefs and values do they have that run counter to the writer? Does the writer adequately address these issues?

4. How well does the writer connect with the audience (sympathetic to their perspective/values)?
   ___ extremely well ___ strong connection ___ does not offend ___ alienates a bit

   The writer attempts to establish common ground with the audience when . . .
   The writer distances himself/herself from the audience when . . .
   The writer could connect better with the audience by . . .

5. The writer uses unemotional, calm, unprejudicial language
   ___ always ___ mostly ___ sometimes ___ seldom

   Examples of calm, unprejudicial language
   Examples of insensitive language

6. The writer acknowledges the reader's merits when . . .

7. What reasons does the writer give for his/her argument? Are they logical and compelling?

8. What evidence does the writer give for the reasons? Is the evidence accurate and sufficient?

9. Are the reasons given directed toward the defined audience?

10. The writer presents balanced arguments, acknowledging their good points and admitting weaknesses in his/her own arguments when . . .

11. What arguments of the audience does the writer acknowledge (and counter)? What arguments of the audience does the writer fail to acknowledge or counter effectively?

Practice Exercises

Exercise 1 Design a think/pair/share writing exercise for a topic in your discipline.

Exercise 2 Prepare a lecture during which students are required to write for 1–3 minutes at the beginning, middle, and end of class.

Exercise 3 Create a question for your class that would require students to summarize in one sentence a concept, process, or reading assignment.

Exercise 4 Create a question that requires students to write a paragraph that explains in their own words a concept or process related to your discipline.

Exercise 5 Create a directed reading assignment that requires more than one level of thinking skills to complete the assignment.

Exercise 6 Decide what assessment strategies would be required for each of the above writing assignments.

Questions for Reflection

1. What writing assignments would help your students develop the abilities you expect of them in your course or at your experiential site?
2. What specific expressive writing assignment topics would be most beneficial for your students?
3. What specific transactional writing assignment topics would be most beneficial for your students?
4. In your teaching modules or clinical experiences, how could you use writing to encourage students to explore attitudes, habits, and values related to the provision of pharmaceutical care?
5. Can you create a writing assignment targeted to specific learning outcomes along with associated criteria and assessment forms?
6. What are the barriers to incorporating writing to learn assignments into your course or at your experiential site?
7. How can you overcome the barriers?

Questions for Planning

This book is meant to be an *orientation* to teaching. Hopefully, it has helped to establish bearings, point to some destinations, and provide some landmarks along the way. What is important now is reflect, internalize, and plan the next steps toward becoming a successful teacher. Here are some questions to begin the process:

1. What, in your opinion, are the criteria for being a successful teacher?
2. What are your strengths relative to these criteria?

3. What criteria would you like most to improve?
4. Can you create a plan for developing the knowledge, skills, attitudes, and values required to be a successful teacher?
5. What are your immediate goals to help students develop critical thinking and problem-solving skills?
6. What are your immediate goals to develop an outcomes-based approach to education?
7. What mentors/resources are available to you in this process?

Notes

1. American Association of Colleges of Pharmacy. Background Paper II: Entry-Level, Curricular Outcomes, Curricular Content and Educational Process [1990]. Commission to Implement Change in Pharmaceutical Education. Am J Pharm Educ 1993;57:377-85.
2. The dynamic relationship between thought and language is extremely complex and controversial. The perspective taken here is related to Vygotsky, LS. In Hanfmann E, Vakar G, ed. and trans. Thought and language. Cambridge, MA: MIT Press, 1965.
3. Smith RE. Unleash the greatness. President-elect Address, Association of American Colleges of Pharmacy, Boston, July 5, 1999. Am J Pharm Educ 1999;63:436-41. See also, Zlatic T. Integrating Education: Chair Report of the 1999/2000 Academic Affairs Committee. Am J Pharm Educ 2000;64:8S-15S.
4. The discussion below is based upon ideas published in a number of works by Walter J. Ong. Particularly relevant here is Orality and literacy: the technologizing of the word. New York: Methuen, 1982.
5. Following the lead of Ernest L. Boyer, the definition of scholarship in higher education has been expanded. Normally, still, scholarly activity must include reflection, dissemination, and assessment, all of which most commonly take place in the form of writing. See Boyer EL. Scholarship reconsidered: priorities of the professoriate. Princeton, NJ: The Carnegie Foundation for the Advancement of Teaching, 1991; and Zlatic TD. Whoa—why did I say I'd do this? Some thoughts on humanities scholarship in pharmacy education. Am J Pharm Educ 1992;56:417-21.
6. Bean JC. Engaging ideas: the professor's guide to integrating writing, critical thinking, and active learning in the classroom. San Francisco: Jossey-Bass, 1996:22-4.
7. In fact, many writing instructors themselves have downplayed or even abandoned mechanics and grammar, sometimes to "liberate" students from confining conventions and sometimes denouncing this fixation with grammatical "correctness" as ideological manifestations of racism, sexism, and classism.
8. For background on the writing-to-learn movement, see Britton J. Language and learning. New York: Penguin Books, 1970; Emig J. Writing as a mode of learning. College Composition and Communication 1977;28:122-8; Fulwiler T. Teaching with writing. Portsmouth, NH: Boynton/Cook Publishers, 1987. For a "brief history of writing to learn in the content areas," see Keys CW. Revitalizing instruction in scientific genres: connecting knowledge production with writing to learn in science. Sci Educ. 1999;83:115-30.
9. Tuana N, ed. Feminism and science. Bloomington: Indiana University Press, 1989. In Gates BT, Shteir AB, eds. Natural eloquence: women reinscribe science. Madison: University of Wisconsin Press, 1997. Maynard M, ed. Science and the construction of women. London: UCL Press, 1997. Belenky M, Clinchy B, Goldberger N, Tarule J. Women's ways of knowing: the development of self, voice, and mind. New York: Basic Books, 1986.

10. For examples, see Strauss M, Fulwiler T. Writing to learn in large lecture classes. J Coll Sci Teach 1989/90;13:158-63. Angelo TM, Cross KP. Classroom assessment techniques: a handbook for college teachers. 2nd ed. San Francisco: Jossey-Bass, 1993. Bean JC. Engaging ideas: the professor's guide to integrating writing, critical thinking, and active learning in the classroom. San Francisco: Jossey-Bass, 1996. Hobson E, Schafermeyer KW. Writing and critical thinking: Writing-to-learn in large classes. Am J Pharm Educ 1994;58:423-7.

11. Bean J, Drenk D, Lee FD. Microtheme strategies for developing cognitive skills. In Griffen CW, ed. Teaching writing in all disciplines. San Francisco: Jossey-Bass, 1982:27-38.

12. Rivard P. A review of writing to learn in science: implications for practice and research. J Res Sci Teach 1994; 31:976; Holiday WG, Yore LD, Alvermann DE. The reading-science learning-writing connection: breakthroughs, barriers, promises. J Res Sci Teach 1994;1:885. Keys CW. Revitalizing instruction in scientific genres: connecting knowledge production with writing to learn in science. Sci Educ 1999;83:116.

13. Schrödinger E. Science and humanism: physics in our time. Cambridge: Cambridge University Press, 1951:7-8.

14. See Ong WJ. The presence of the word: some prolegomena for cultural and religious history. New York: Simon and Shuster, 1967, 35-53. Eisenstein EL. The printing press as an agent of change: Communications and cultural transformations in early-modern Europe. Cambridge: Cambridge University Press, 1979.

15. Luke A. Introduction. In Halliday MAK, Martin JR. Writing science: literacy and discursive power. Pittsburgh: University of Pittsburgh Press, 1993, xii.

16. Halliday MAK, Martin JR. Writing science: Literacy and discursive power. Pittsburgh: University of Pittsburgh Press, 1993, 8.

17. The emergence of electronic communications technology and its potential implications for human thought and expression provide for tantalizing speculations regarding the evolution of writing and research in the upcoming century. Just as the printing press contributed to the development of scientific thinking and language, electronic communication technology will likely influence new patterns of thought and writing. For some preliminary analyses, see Heim M. Electric language: A philosophical study of word processing. New Haven: Yale University Press, 1987. Bolter JD. Writing space: the computer, hypertext, and the history of writing. Hillsdale, NJ: Lawrence Erlbaum, 1991. Lanham RA. The electronic word: democracy, technology, and the arts. Chicago: University of Chicago Press, 1993. Welch KE. Electric rhetoric: Classical rhetoric, oralism, and a new literacy. Cambridge, MA: The MIT Press, 1999.

18. Keys CW. Revitalizing instruction in scientific genres: connecting knowledge production with writing to learn in science. Sci Educ 1999;83:121.

19. For an overview in the sciences, see Rivard, 969-983. Examples of general strategies for writing in the sciences can be found in Glynn SM, Muth KD. Reading and writing to learn science: achieving scientific literacy. J Res Sci Teach 1994;31:1057-73. For more tempered results, see Schumacher GM, Gradwohl J. Conceptualizing and measuring knowledge change due to writing. Res Teach English 1991;67-96.

20. Aspinwall L, Miller LD. Students' reliance on writing as a process to learn first semester calculus. J Instr Psych 1997;24(4):253-61.

21. Van Orden N. Is writing an effective way to learn chemical concepts? J Chem Educ 1987;67:583-5.

22. Wilson JW. Writing to learn in an organic chemistry class. J Chem Educ. 1994;71:1019-20.

23. Beins BC. Writing assignments in statistics classes encourage students to learn interpretation. Teach Psych 1993;20:161-4.

24. Moore R. Writing to learn biology. J Coll Sci Teach 1994;23(5):289-95.

25. Allen DG, Bowers B, Diekelmann N. Writing to learn: a reconceptualization of thinking and writing in the nursing curriculum. J Nurs Educ 1989;28:6-11. See also, McCarthy DO. Implementation of writing-to-learn in a program of nursing. Nurse Educ 1994;19:32-5.

26. Holiday-Goodman M, Lively BT, Nemire R, Mullin J. Development of a teaching module on written and verbal communication skills. Am J Pharm Educ 1994;58:257-62. See also Holiday-Goodman M, Lively BT. Writing across the curriculum for colleges of pharmacy: a source book. Toledo, OH: The University of Toledo College of Pharmacy and American Association of Colleges of Pharmacy, 1992. And see Hobson EH. Writing across the pharmacy curriculum: an annotated bibliography. J Pharm Teach 1996;5:37-54.

27. Zlatic TD, Nowak DM, Sylvester D. Integrating general and professional education through a study of herbal products: An intercollegiate collaboration. Am J Pharm Educ 2000;64:83-94.

28. Prosser TR, Burke JM, Hobson EH. Teaching pharmacy students to write in the medical record. Am J Pharm Educ 1997;61:136-40.

29. For service learning within pharmacy, see Nickman NA (Re-)learning to care: use of service-learning as an early professionalization experience. Am J Pharm Educ 1998;62:380-7.

30. Two examples of expressive writing from the medical literature are: Poirier S, Ahrens WR, Brauner DJ. Songs of innocence and experience: students' poems about their medical education. Acad Med 1998;73:473-8; and Deloney LA, Carey M J, Geeman HG. Using electronic journal writing to foster reflection and provide feedback in an introduction to clinical medicine. Acad Med 1998;73(5):574-5.

31. Writing emphasis or writing intensive courses employ writing to learn principles and strategies for students to learn a subject matter. Usually such a course requires a minimum number of written pages (often 20-40 pages), a number of different writing assignments (often three to six), and the rewriting of two or three of those assignments after receiving feedback from self, peers, and instructor. For the efficacy of such a writing emphasis course in pharmacy, see Ranelli P and Nelson JV. Assessing writing perceptions and practices of pharmacy students. Am J Pharm Educ 1998;62:426-32.

Works Cited

Abate MA, Stamatakis MK, Haggett RR. Excellence in curriculum development and assessment. Am J Pharm Educ 2003;67(3):Article 89.

Abate MA, Meyer-Stout PJ, Stamatakis MK, Gannett PM, Dunsworth TS, Nardi AH. Development and evaluation of computerized problem-based learning cases emphasizing basic sciences concepts. Am J Pharm Educ 2000;64:74-82.

Adamcik B, Hurley S, Erramouspe J. Assessment of pharmacy students' critical thinking and problem-solving abilities. Am J Pharm Educ 1996;60:256-65.

Allen DD, Bond CA. Prepharmacy predictors of success in pharmacy school: grade point averages, pharmacy college admissions test, communication abilities, and critical thinking skills. Pharmacotherapy 2001;21(7):842-9.

Allen DG, Bowers B, Diekelmann N. Writing to learn: a reconceptualization of thinking and writing in the nursing curriculum. J Nurs Educ 1989;28(1):6-11.

Alverno College. Ability-based learning program (Rev. ed.). Milwaukee, WI: Alverno College Institute, 1994.

Alverno College. Student assessment-as-learning at Alverno College. Milwaukee, WI: Alverno College Institute, 1994.

American Association of Colleges of Pharmacy. Background paper I: what is the mission of pharmaceutical education? [1990]. Am J Pharm Educ1993;57:374-6.

American Association of Colleges of Pharmacy. Background Paper II: Entry-Level, Curricular Outcomes, Curricular Content and Educational Process [1990]. Commission to Implement Change in Pharmaceutical Education. Am J Pharm Educ 1993;57:377-85.

American Association of Colleges of Pharmacy. Educational outcomes. Center for the Advancement of Pharmaceutical Education (CAPE). Alexandria, VA: American Association of Colleges of Pharmacy, 1994.

American Association of Colleges of Pharmacy. Educational outcomes. Center for the Advancement of Pharmaceutical Education (CAPE). Alexandria, VA: American Association of Colleges of Pharmacy, 2004.

Anderson JR. Cognitive psychology and its implications. San Francisco: Freeman, 1980.

Angelo TM, Cross KP. Classroom assessment techniques: a handbook for college teachers. 2nd ed. San Francisco: Jossey-Bass, 1993.

Armstrong T. Multiple intelligences in the classroom. Alexandria, VA: Association for Supervision and Curriculum Development, 1994.

Arons AB. A guide to introductory physics teaching. New York: John Wiley and Sons, 1990.

Aspinwall L., Miller LD. Students' reliance on writing as a process to learn first semester calculus. J Instr Psych 1997;24(4):253-61.

Association of American Colleges. Integrity in the college curriculum: a report to the academic community. Project on Redefining the Meaning and Purpose of Baccalaureate Degrees. Washington DC: Association of American Colleges, 1985.

Association of American Colleges and Universities. Taking responsibility for the quality of the baccalaureate degree: a report from the greater expectations project on accreditation and assessment. Washington DC: Association of American Colleges and Universities, 2004.

Austin Z, Boyd C. Development of a sequenced strategic thinking assignment syllabus for a senior-level professional practice course. Am J Pharm Educ 1998;62:119-23.

Austin Z. Development and validation of the pharmacists' inventory of learning styles (PILS). Am J Pharm Educ 2004;68:article 37.

Banta T, Lund J, Black K, Oblander F, eds. Making a difference: outcomes of a decade of assessment in higher education. San Francisco: Jossey-Bass, 1993.

Barr RB, Tagg J. From teaching to learning: a new paradigm for undergraduate education. Change 1995;27:12-25.

Barrows HS. How to design a problem-based curriculum for the preclinical years. New York: Springer, 1985.

Bean J, Drenk D, Lee FD. Microtheme strategies for developing cognitive skills. Griffen CW, ed. Teaching writing in all disciplines. San Francisco: Jossey-Bass, 1982:27-38.

Bean JC. Engaging ideas: the professor's guide to integrating writing, critical thinking, and active learning in the classroom. San Francisco: Jossey-Bass, 1996.

Becker ES, Schafermeyer KW. Educational care 101: prerequisite for pharmaceutical care. J Pharm Teach 1993:3:3-14.

Beins BC. Writing assignments in statistics classes encourage students to learn interpretation. Teach Psych 1993;20:161-4.

Belenky M, Clinchy B, Goldberger NR, Tarule JM. Women's ways of knowing: the development of self, voice, and mind. New York: Basic Books, 1986.

Berger BA. Communication skills for pharmacists: building relationships, improving care. 2nd ed. Washington DC, American Pharmacists Association, 2005.

Berner ES. Paradigms and problem-solving: a literature review. J Med Educ 1984:59(8):625-33.

Bloom BS, Hastings JT, Madaus GF. Handbook on formative and summative valuation of student learning. New York: McGraw-Hill, 1971.

Boh LE, Pitterle ME, Wiederholt JB, Tyler LS. Development and application of a computer simulation program to enhance the clinical problem-solving skills of students. Am J Pharm Educ 1987;51:253-61.

Boice R. Advice for new faculty members: nihil nimus. Boston: Allyn and Bacon, 2000.

Bolter JD. Writing space: the computer, hypertext, and the history of writing. Hillsdale, NJ: Lawrence Erlbaum, 1991.

Bonwell CC, Eison AJ. Active learning: creating excitement in the classroom. ASHE-ERIC Higher Education Report No. 1. Washington DC: George Washington University, 1991.

Bonwell CC. The enhanced lecture: a resource book for faculty. Cape Girardeau: MO: The Center for Teaching and Learning, Southeast Missouri State University, 1991.

Bootman JL, Garnett WR, Miller WA, Ryan MR, Spratto GR. Components of a minimum college curriculum: relationship to pharmacy education. White paper from the 1985-86 Academic Affairs Committee. Am J Pharm Educ 1986;50:386-9.

Boud D, Feletti G, eds. The challenge of problem based learning. New York: St. Martin's Press, 1991.

Boyer EL. Scholarship reconsidered: priorities of the professoriate. Princeton, NJ: The Carnegie Foundation for the Advancement of Teaching, 1991.

Britton J. Language and learning. New York: Penguin Books, 1970.

Busto U, Knight K, Janecek E, Isaac P, Parker K. A problem-based learning course for pharmacy students on alcohol and psychoactive substance abuse disorders. Am J Pharm Educ 1994;58:55-60.

Carraccio C, Wolfsthal SD, Englander R, Ferentz K, Martin C. Shifting paradigms: From Flexner to competencies. Acad Med 2002;77(5): 385-91.

Catney CM., Currie JD. Implementing problem-based learning with WWW support in an introductory pharmaceutical care course. Am J Pharm Educ 1999;63:97-104.

Chalmers R, Grotpeter J, Hollenbeck G, Nickman N, Sommi R, Zlatic T. Changing to an outcome-based, assessment guided curriculum: a report of the Focus Group on Liberalization of the Professional Curriculum. Am J Pharm Educ 1994;58:108-15.

Chalmers RK, Gibson RD, Schumacher GE, Sorby DL, Zografi G. Liberal education—a key structural component in pharmacy education. Report of the 1986-1987 Argus Commission. Am J Pharm Educ 1987;51:446-50.

Chalmers RK, Grotpeter JJ, Hollenbeck RG, et al. Ability-based outcome goals for the professional curriculum: a report of the Focus Group on Liberalization of the Professional Curriculum. Am J Pharm Educ 1992;56:304-9.

Chalmers RK. Pharmacy education strategy: the solution is in the problem. Am J Pharm Educ 1988;52:388-93.

Cisneros RM, Salisbury-Glennon JD, Anderson-Harper HM. Status of problem-based learning research in pharmacy education: a call for future research. Am J Pharm Educ 2002;66:19-26.

Cohen JL. Chair Report for the Academic Affairs Committee. Am J Pharm Educ 1988; 52:409-11.

Cooper JL, Robinson P, McKinney M. Cooperative Learning in the Classroom. In Halpern, DF, ed. Changing college classrooms: new teaching and learning strategies for an increasingly complex world. San Francisco: Jossey-Bass, 1994.

Culbertson VL, Kale M, Jarvi EJ. Problem-based learning: a tutorial model incorporating pharmaceutical diagnosis. Am J Pharm Educ 1997;61:18-26.

Davidson N, Worsham T, eds. Enhancing thinking through cooperative learning. New York: Teachers College Press, 1992.

Delafuente JC, Munyer TO, Angaran DM, Doering PL. A problem solving active-learning course in pharmacotherapy. Am J Pharm Educ 1994;58(1):61-4.

Deloney LA, Carey MJ, Geeman HG. Using electronic journal writing to foster reflection and provide feedback in an introduction to clinical medicine. Acad Med 1998;73(5):574-5.

Des Marchais JE, Dumais B. Issues in implementing a problem-based learning curriculum at the University of Sherbrooke. Annals of Community-Oriented Education 1990;3:9-23.

Donovan MS, Bransford JD, Pellegrino JW, eds. How people learn: bridging research and practice. National Research Council. Washington DC: National Academy Press, 1999.

Dumbleton SM, Soleau JK. Liberal studies and the pharmacy curriculum: the importance of integration. Am J Pharm Educ 1991;55:59-64.

Eck JC. Assessing and researching problem-based learning. Birmingham, AL: Samford University Press, 2002.

Eisenstein EL. The printing press as an agent of change: communications and cultural transformations in early-modern Europe. Cambridge: Cambridge University Press, 1979.

Emig, J. Writing as a mode of learning. College Composition and Communication. 1977;28:122-8.

Ennis RH. A concept of critical thinking. Harv Educ Review 1962;32:81-111.

Epstein RM, Hundert EM. Defining and Assessing Professional Competence. JAMA. 2002;287:226-35.

Facione PA. Critical thinking: a statement of expert consensus for purposes of educational assessment and instruction. Washington DC: U.S. Department of Education, Office of Education Research and Improvement, 1990.

Fadiman A. The spirit catches you and you fall down: a Hmong child, her American doctors, and the collision of two cultures. New York: Farrar, Straus, and Giroux, 1997.

Filene PG. The joy of teaching: a practical guide for new college instructors. Chapel Hill: University of North Carolina Press, 2005.

Fisher RC. The potential for problem-based learning in pharmacy education: a clinical therapeutics course in diabetes. Am J Pharm Educ 1994;58(2):183-9.

Fulwiler T. Teaching with writing. Portsmouth, NH: Boynton/Cook Publishers, 1987.

Gardner H. Intelligence reframed: multiple intelligence for the 21st century. New York: Basic Books, 1999.

Gardner H. Multiple intelligences: a theory in practice. New York: Basic Books, 1993.

Gates BT, Shteir AB, eds. Natural eloquence: women reinscribe science. Madison: University of Wisconsin Press, 1997.

Glynn SM, Muth KD. Reading and writing to learn science: achieving scientific literacy. J Res Sci Teach 1994;31:1057-73.

Goodsell AS, Maher MR, Tinto V, Smith BL, McGregor J. Collaborative learning: a sourcebook for higher education. University Park, PA: National Center on Postsecondary Education, 1992.

Gregory MW. Critical thinking and liberal education. Perspectives 1988;18:9-25.

Hafferty FW, Franks R. The hidden curriculum, ethics teaching, and the structure of medical education. Acad Med 1994:69:861-71.

Hafler JP. Case writing: case writers' perspectives, in Boud D and Feletti G, eds. The challenge of problem based learning. New York: St. Martin's Press, 1991:150-8.

Halliday MAK, Martin JR. Writing science: Literacy and discursive power. Pittsburgh: University of Pittsburgh Press, 1993.

Harris FK, Harrold MW, Giudici RA, et al. Development and implementation of critical thinking assignments throughout a pharmacy curriculum. Am J Pharm Educ 1997;61:1-11.

Hartzema AG. Teaching therapeutic reasoning through the case-study approach: adding the probabilistic dimension. Am J Pharm Educ 1994;58:436-40.

Haworth IS, Bolger MB, Eriksen SP. The use of computer-based case studies in a problem-solving curriculum. Am J Pharm Educ 1997;61:97-102.

Haworth IS, Eriksen SP, Chmait SH, et al. Use of computer-based case studies in a problem-solving curriculum. Am J Pharm Educ 1997;61:97-102.

Haworth IS, Eriksen SP, Chmait, SH, et al. A problem based learning case study approach to pharmaceutics: faculty and student perspectives. Am J Pharm Educ 1998;62:398-405.

Hawthorne EM. Case study and critical thinking. Issues and Inquiry in College Learning and Teaching.1991:60-1.

Heim M. Electric language: A philosophical study of word processing. New Haven: Yale University Press, 1987.

Hobson EH, Schafermeyer KW. Writing and critical thinking: Writing-to-learn in large classes. Am J Pharm Educ 1994;58:423-7.

Hobson EH. Writing across the pharmacy curriculum: an annotated bibliography. J Pharm Teach 1996;5:37-54.

Holiday WG, Yore LD, Alvermann DE. The reading-science learning-writing connection: breakthroughs, barriers, promises. J Res Sci Teach 1994;1:885.

Holiday-Goodman M, Lively BT. Writing across the curriculum for colleges of pharmacy: a source book. Toledo, OH: The University of Toledo College of Pharmacy and American Association of Colleges of Pharmacy, 1992.

Holiday-Goodman M, Lively BT, Nemire R, Mullin J. Development of a teaching module on written and verbal communication skills. Am J Pharm Educ 1994;58:257-62.

Holmes RL. The limited relevance of analytical ethics to the problems of bioethics. J Med Philos 1990;15:143-59.

Hunter KA. Poster presentations: an alternative to the traditional classroom lecture. Am J Pharm Educ 1997;61:78-80.

Institute of Medicine. Crossing the quality chasm: a new health system for the 21st century. Washington DC: The National Academy Press, 2001.

Institute of Medicine. Greiner AC, Knebel E, eds. Health professions education: a bridge to quality. Washington DC: The National Academies Press, 2003.

Institute of Medicine. To err is human: building a safer health system. Washington DC: The National Academy Press, 2001.

Jang R, Solad SW. Teaching pharmacy students problem-solving: theory and present status. Am J Pharm Educ 1990;54:161-6.

Joint Commission of Pharmacy Practitioners. Future vision of pharmacy practice. In Maine LL. The class of 2015. Am J Pharm Educ 2005;69(3):article 56.

Kane MP, Briceland LL, Hamilton RA. Solving drug-related problems in the professional experience program. Am J Pharm Educ 1993;57:347-51.

Karplus R. Science teaching and the development of reasoning. Berkeley, CA: University of California, 1977.

Kaufman DM, Mann KV. Students' perceptions about their courses in problem-based-learning and conventional curricula. Acad Med 1996:71:s52-s54.

Keys CW. Revitalizing instruction in scientific genres: connecting knowledge production with writing to learn in science. Sci Educ 1999;83:115-30.

Kiewra KA, DuBois NF, Christian D, McShane A, Meyerhoffer M, Roskelley D. Note-taking functions and techniques. J Educ Psych 1991;83:240-5.

King A. Inquiry as a tool in critical thinking. In Halpern DF, ed. Changing college classrooms. San Francisco: Jossey-Bass, 1994:13-38.

Kolb DA. Experiential learning: experience as the source of learning and development. Englewood Cliffs, NJ: Prentice Hall, 1984.

Kremers E. Proceedings of the American Conference of Pharmaceutical Faculties at the Fourth Annual Meeting, 1903. Cited in Newcomer J, Bunnell KP, McGrath EJ. Liberal education and pharmacy. New York: Institute of Higher Education, Columbia University, 1960.

Kurfiss JG. Critical thinking: theory, research, practice, and possibilities. ASHE-ERIC Higher Education Report No. 2. College Station, TX: Association for the Study of Higher Education, Texas A&M University, 1988.

Lanham RA. The electronic word: democracy, technology, and the arts. Chicago: University of Chicago Press, 1993.

Lawson AE. The reality of general cognitive operations. Sci Educ 1982;66:229-41.
lbanese MA, Mitchell S. Problem-based learning: a review of literature on its outcomes and implementation issues. Acad Med 1993;68(1):52-81.

Loacker G, Cromwell L, Fey J, Rutherford D. Analysis and Communication at Alverno: an approach to critical thinking. Milwaukee, WI: Alverno Productions, 1984.

Lowman J. Mastering the techniques of teaching. San Francisco: Jossey-Bass, 1984.

Lucas CJ, Murry JW Jr. New faculty: a practical guide for academic beginners. New York: Palgrave, 2002.

Luke A. Introduction. In Halliday MAK, Martin JR. Writing science: literacy and discursive power. Pittsburgh: University of Pittsburgh Press, 1993.

Lush RM III, McAuley JM, Kroboth PD. Experimental design for clinical research: a student-centered problem-based approach. Am J Pharm Educ 1993;57:39-43.

Maddux M. Institutionalizing assessment as learning within an ability-based program. In Wilkins, NE, ed. Handbook for pharmacy educators: Contemporary teaching principles and strategies. New York: Haworth Press, 2000: 141-60.

Maine LL. CAPE outcomes 2004: What do pharmacists do? Am J Pharm Educ 2004;68(3):article 78.

Maynard M, ed. Science and the construction of women. London: UCL Press, 1997.

McCarthy DO. Implementation of writing-to-learn in a program of nursing. Nurse Educ 1994;19:32-5.

McKeachie WJ, Pintrich PR, Lin Y, Smith DAF. Teaching and learning in the college classroom. Ann Arbor: University of Michigan, 1986.

McPeck JE. Critical thinking and education. New York: St. Martin's Press, 1981.

McPeck JE. Stalking beasts, but swatting flies: the teaching of critical thinking. Can J Educ 1984;93:28-44.

Mehvar, R. Development and evaluation of quasi problem-based objective-driven learning strategy in introductory and clinical pharmacokinetic courses. Am J Pharm Educ 1999;7:17-27.

Mentkowski M and Associates. Learning that lasts: integrating learning, development, and performance in college and beyond. San Francisco: Jossey-Bass, 2000.

Meyer SP, Popovich NG. Experience and observations about the guided design instructional methodology. Am J Pharm Educ 1990;54:35-9.

Meyers C. Teaching students to think critically. San Francisco: Jossey-Bass 1986, 26-39.

Miller DR. An assessment of critical thinking: can pharmacy students evaluate clinical studies like experts? Am J Pharm Educ 2004;68:article 5.

Miller DR. Longitudinal assessment of critical thinking in pharmacy students. Am J Pharm Educ 2003;67:article 120.

Monk-Tutor MR. Overview of MSOP curriculum and adoption of PBL. PBL Insight. 2003;6(1).

Monaghan MS, Vanderbush RE, McKay AB, Gardner SF, Schneider EF. A computerized database approach to enhance critical thinking. J Pharm Teach 1999;7:35-50.

Moore R. Writing to learn biology. J Coll Sci Teach 1994;23(5):289-95.

Murawski MM, Muraski D, Wilson M. Service-learning and pharmaceutical education: an exploratory survey. Am J Pharm Educ 1999;63:160-4.

Nelson CE. Skewered on the unicorn's horn: the illusion of tragic tradeoff between content and critical thinking in the teaching of science. In Crow LW, ed. Enhancing critical thinking in the sciences. Washington DC: Society for College Science Teachers, 1989.

Newcomer J, Bunnell K, McGrath E. Liberal education and pharmacy. New York: Institute of Higher Learning, Columbia University, 1960.

Newton GD, Popovich NG, Lehman JD. Development and evaluation of computer-assisted guided design for problem-solving instruction in self-care pharmacy practice. Am J Pharm Educ 1991;55:301-10.

Newton GD, Tracy TS, Popovich NG. The development and implementation of an integrating pharmacy practice laboratory. Am J Pharm Educ 1990;4:138-45.

Nickman NA. (Re-)learning to care: use of service-learning as an early professionalization experience. Am J of Pharm Ed. 1998;62:380-7.

Nii LJ, Chin AA. Comparative trial of problem-based learning versus didactic lectures on clerkship performance. Am J Pharm Educ 1996;60(2):162-4.

Odedina FT, Clemmons CD, Dukes N. Mulifaceted active learning approach to teaching pharmacy health care and behavior Am J Pharm Educ 2000;65:276-83.

Ong WJ. Presidential address 1978: the human nature of professionalism. PMLA 1979;94:385-94.

Ong WJ. The presence of the word: some prolegomena for cultural and religious history. New York: Simon and Shuster, 1967.

Ong WJ. Orality and literacy: the technologizing of the word. New York: Methuen, 1982.

Palmer PJ. The courage to teach: exploring the inner landscape of a teacher's life. San Francisco: Jossey-Bass Publishers, 1998.

Palomba CA, Banta TW. Assessment essentials: planning, implementing and improving assessment in higher education. San Francisco: Jossey-Bass, 1999.

Parrish E. Proceedings of the American Pharmaceutical Association at the Twentieth Annual Meeting, 1872. Cited in Newcomer J, Bunnell KP, McGrath EJ. Liberal education and pharmacy. New York: Institute of Higher Education, Columbia University, 1960.

Paul R. Critical thinking: what every person needs to survive in a rapidly changing world. Rohnert Park, CA: Center for Critical Thinking and Moral Critique, 1990.

Pawlak SM. Development and validation of guided design scenarios for problem-solving instruction. Am J Pharm Educ 1989;53:7-16.

Perrier D, Winslade N, Pugsley J, Lavack L, Strand L. Designing a pharmaceutical care curriculum. Am J Pharm Educ 1995;59:113-24.

Perry WG Jr. Forms of intellectual and ethical development in the college years: a scheme. New York: Holt, Rinehart, 1970.

Phillips CR, Chesnut RJ, Rospond RM. The California critical thinking instruments for benchmarking, program assessment, and directing curricular change. Am J Pharm Educ 2004;68:article 101.

Piper B, DeYoung M, Lamsam G. Student perceptions of a service-learning experience. Am J Pharm Educ 2000;64:159-65.

Poirier S, Ahrens WR, Brauner DJ. Songs of innocence and experience: students' poems about their medical education. Acad Med 1998;73:473-78.

Popovich NG. The educational care of pharmacy. Am J Pharm Educ 1991;55:349-55.

Presseisen BZ. Thinking skills: research and practice. Washington DC: National Education Association, 1986.

Prosser TR, Burke JM, Hobson EH. Teaching pharmacy students to write in the medical record. Am J Pharm Educ 1997;61:136-40.

Pungente MD, Wasan KM, Moffett C. Using learning styles to evaluate first-year pharmacy students' preferences toward different activities associated with the problem-based learning approach. Am J Pharm Educ 2003;66:119-24.

Purkerson D, Mason H, Chalmers R, Popovich G, Scott S. Expansion of ability-based education using an assessment center approach with pharmacists as assessors. Am J Pharm Educ 1997;61:241-8.

Purkerson D, Mason H, Chalmers R, Popovich G, Scott S. Evaluating pharmacy students' ability-based educational outcomes using an assessment center approach. Am J Pharm Educ 1996;60:239-48.

Raisch DW, Holdsworth MT, Mann PL, Kabat H. Incorporating problem-based, student-centered learning into pharmacy externship rotations. Am J Pharm Educ 1995;59:265-72.

Ranelli P, Nelson JV. Assessing writing perceptions and practices of pharmacy students. Am J Pharm Educ 1998;62:426-32.

Rangachari PK. Design of a problem-based undergraduate course in pharmacology: implications for the teaching of physiology. Am J Physiol 1991;260:S14-S21.

Regal PJ. The anatomy of judgment. Minneapolis: University of Minnesota Press, 1990.

Reich WT. What care can mean for pharmaceutical ethics. J Pharm Teach 1996;5:1-17.

Reinsmith WA. Archetypal forms in teaching: a continuum. New York: Greenwood Press, 1992.

Rhodes DG. A practical approach to problem-based learning: simple technology makes PBL accessible. Am J Pharm Educ 1999;63:410-4.

Rivard P. A review of writing to learn in science: implications for practice and research. J Res Sci Teach 1994;31:976.

Robertson KE, McDaniel AM. Interdisciplinary professional education: a collaborative clinical teaching project. Am. J Pharm Educ 1995;59:131-6.

Ruhl KL, Hughes CA, Schloss PJ. Using the pause procedure to enhance lecture recall. Teacher Educ and Special Educ 1987;10:14-8.

Sajé N. Teaching for tips. Liberal Educ 2005;91:48-51.

Salamon LB. Integrity in the pharmacy curriculum. Am J Pharm Educ 1985;49:361-70.

Schrödinger E. Science and humanism: physics in our time. Cambridge: Cambridge University Press, 1951.

Schumacher GM, Gradwohl J. Conceptualizing and measuring knowledge change due to writing. Res Teach Eng 1991;67-96.

Shuck AA, Phillips CR. Assessing pharmacy students' learning styles and personality types: A ten-year analysis. Am J Pharm Educ 1999;63:27-33.

Shulman LS. Professing the liberal arts. In Orrill R, ed. Education and democracy: re-imagining liberal learning in America. New York: The College Board, 1997.

Sibbald D. Innovative, problem-based, pharmaceutical care courses for self-medication. Am J Pharm Educ 1998;62:109-19.

Sims PJ. Utilizing the peer group method with case studies to teach pharmacokinetics. Am J Pharm Educ 1994;58:73-7.

Smith RE. Unleash the greatness. President-Elect Address, Association of American Colleges of Pharmacy, Boston, July 5, 1999. Am J Pharm Ed 1999; 63(4):436-41.

Spiro H. What is empathy and can it be taught? Ann Intern Med. 1992;116:843-6.

Stark JS, Lowther MA. Exploring common ground in liberal and professional education. New directions for teaching and learning 1989;40:7-20.

Stark JS, Lowther MA. Strengthening the ties that bind: integrating undergraduate liberal and professional study. Report of the Professional Preparation Network. Ann Arbor, MI: University of Michigan, 1988.

Stevens DD, Levi A. Introduction to rubrics: an assessment tool to save grading time, convey effective feedback, and promote student learning. Sterling, VA: Stylus, 2005.

Stonewater JL. Strategies for problem solving. In Young RE, ed. Fostering critical thinking. San Francisco: Jossey-Bass, 1980, 33-43.

Strand LM, Morley PC. A problem-based student-centered approach to pharmacy education. Am J Pharm Educ 1987;51:75-9.

Strand LM, Morley PC. Evolving health care systems: academic implications for teaching methodologies with emphasis on administration and practice. Am J Pharm Educ 1987;51:402-6.

Strauss M, Fulwiler T. Writing to learn in large lecture classes. J Coll Sci Teach 1989/90;13:158-63.

Sutherland T, Bonwell CC, eds. Using active learning in college classes: a range of options for faculty. San Francisco, CA: Jossey-Bass, 1996.

Swanson DB, Case SM, van der Vleuten CPM. Strategies for student assessment. In Boud D and Feletti G, eds. The challenge of problem based learning. New York: St. Martin's Press, 1991:260-73.

Tuana N, ed. Feminism and science. Bloomington: Indiana University Press, 1989.

Turner CJ, Altiere R, Clark L, Maffeo C, Valdez C. Competency-based introductory pharmacy practice experiential courses. Am J Pharm Educ 2005;69(2):article 21.

Van Berkel HJM. Assessment in a problem-based medical curriculum. Higher Educ 1990;19(2):123-46.

VanOrden N. Is writing an effective way to learn chemical concepts? J Chem Educ 1987;67:583-5.

Vrahnos D, Dahdal W, Zlatic T, Maddux M. The peripheral brain: a tool to foster higher-order thinking in abilities-based courses. Am J Pharm Educ 1998;62:44-9.

Vrahnos D, Maddux M. Introductory clinical clerkship during the first and second professional year: emphasis in clinical practice and writing. Am J Pharm Educ 1998;62:53-61.

Vygotsky LS. Thought and language. Hanfmann E, Vakar G, ed and trans. Cambridge, MA: MIT Press, 1965.

Wales CE, Nardi AH. It takes thinking to produce a scholar. Am J Pharm Educ 1988;52(4):385-8.

Wales CE, Nardi AH, Stager RA. Decision making: new paradigm for education. Educ Leadership 1986;43:37-41.

Wales CE, Nardi AH, Stager RH. Professional decision making. Morgantown, WV: Center for Guided Design, West Virginia University, 1986.

Wales CE, Stager RA, Long TR. Guided engineering design. St. Paul, MN: West, 1974.

Wallace C, Franson K. Incorporation of ability-based outcome education into pharmacotherapeutics using an expanded SOAP format. Am J Pharm Educ 1996;60:87-92.

Welch KE. Electric rhetoric: Classical rhetoric, oralism, and a new literacy. Cambridge, MA: MIT Press, 1999.

Whitman N, Schwenk TS. Problem solving in medical education: can it be taught? Curr Surg 1986;43:453-9.

Wilson JW. Writing to learn in an organic chemistry class. J Chem Educ 1994;71:1019-20.

Winslade N. Large group problem-based learning: a revision from traditional to pharmaceutical care-based therapeutics. Am J Pharm Educ 1994;58:64-73.

Woods DR. Problem solving in practice. In Gabel D, ed. Problem solving: what research says to the teacher, Vol. 5. Washington DC: National Science Teachers Association, 1989.

Woods DR. The MPS strategy book. Hamilton, Canada: McMaster University, 1992.

Zellmer WA. Searching for the soul of pharmacy. Am J Health Syst Pharm 1996;53:1911-6.

Zlatic TD, Nowak DM, Sylvester D. Integrating general and professional education through a study of herbal products: An intercollegiate collaboration. Am J Pharm Educ 2000;64:83-94.

Zlatic TD. Abilities-based assessment within pharmacy education: Preparing students for practice of pharmaceutical care. In Wilkins, NE, ed. Handbook for pharmacy educators: Contemporary teaching principles and strategies. New York: Haworth Press, 2000:5-27.

Zlatic TD. Redefining a profession: assessment in pharmacy education. In Palumbo C, Banta T, eds. Assessment of student competence in accredited disciplines: illustrative case studies. Sterling, VA: Stylus Publications, 2001.

Zlatic TD. Integrating education: chair report of the 1999/2000 Academic Affairs Committee, American Association of Colleges of Pharmacy. Am. J Pharm Educ 2000;64:8S-15S.

Zlatic TD. Whoa—why did I say I'd do this? Some thoughts on humanities scholarship in pharmacy education. Am J Pharm Educ 1992;56:417-21.

Index

Abilities: 2, 7, 14-9, 21-22, 28-30, 32, 34, 36, 39, 42-44, 47, 49, 56, 65-66, 68, 70, 77, 81-91, 94, 96, 97, 100-105, 108, 110, 113, 116, 119-120, 128, 133, 145-146
Ability-based education: 12, 23, 39, 45, 82, 103-105, 143
Active learning: 2, 12, 14-15, 18, 22, 39, 51, 56-57, 59, 61-66, 68-69, 71-72, 77-79, 81, 90, 105, 108, 112, 116, 129-130, 134-135, 142, 144
Alverno College: 3, 21-22, 39, 40, 45, 81, 104-105, 133
American Association of Colleges of Pharmacy: 3, 15, 24-25, 27, 44, 64, 78-79, 104, 129, 131, 133, 138, 146
Assessment: 1, 2, 12, 14, 17-18, 24, 29, 33, 36, 40-42, 44-46, 50, 57, 71, 75, 78, 81-85, 87, 89-92, 95-105, 108, 116, 118-121, 124, 126-130, 133-134, 136-137, 140-146
Assessment feedback: 2, 14, 18, 57, 83-90, 92, 96-98, 100-103
Assessment forms: 101-103, 128
Assessment-as-learning: 18, 98-99, 126
Association of American Colleges and Universities: 134
Barr, Robert: 12, 23, 134
Belenky, Mary: 24, 37, 45, 129, 134
Bloom, Benjamin: 34-35, 38, 45, 49, 51-52, 54, 58-59, 83, 90, 115, 135
Bonwell, Charles: 3, 71-2, 77, 79, 105, 135, 144
CAPE Educational Outcomes: 23
Case studies: 18, 41, 44, 64-67, 76, 78-79, 94, 104, 108, 138, 144, 146
Collaborative learning: 62-63, 65-67, 74, 78, 101, 137
Commission to Implement Change in Pharmacy Education: 104
Critical thinking: 3, 16, 18, 27-53, 55-57, 59, 61, 64, 66, 68-71, 78-81, 90, 108, 116, 129-130, 133, 134, 137-142, 144
Facione, Peter: 33, 35, 38, 45, 137
Fiduciary relationships/responsibilities: 6-7
Grading template: 120-121
Group learning: 66, 78
Guided design: 41, 46, 57, 66-67, 78-9, 141-142, 145
Holstad, Sheldon: 3, 105
Institute of Medicine: 12, 23, 25, 139
Integration of general and professional education: 22
Learning paradigm: 12-14, 23, 81
Learning styles: 8, 14, 24, 43, 63, 69, 134, 143-144
Liberalization of the professional curriculum: 17, 24, 45, 104, 136
Loacker, Georgine: 3, 45, 104, 140
Maddux, Michael: 3, 59, 104-105, 140, 145
McPeck, John: 33-34, 45, 59, 140
Mentkowski, Marcia: 21, 104, 141
Multiple intelligences: 24, 28, 134, 137
Nelson, Craig: 28, 37, 45, 131, 141, 143
Objectives: 67, 82-84, 87, 90-91
Ong, Walter: 9, 114, 129-130, 142

Outcomes: 2, 5, 12, 15-18, 21-24, 29-30, 39, 44, 46, 49, 52, 56, 65, 67-70, 78, 81-92, 103-105, 108, 110, 119-121, 128-129, 133-134, 140, 143
Palmer, Parker: 9, 142
Paul, Richard: 32-33, 45-46, 142, 145
Perry, William: 36-37, 45, 49, 142
Pharmaceutical care: 2, 5, 9, 12-16, 19, 21, 30, 49, 50, 59, 67, 78-79, 81-82, 85-86, 88, 94, 104-105, 107, 116-117, 119-120, 128, 134-135, 142, 144, 146
Problem-based learning: 7, 18, 23-24, 41-42, 46, 57, 66-67, 77-79, 108, 133, 135-137, 140, 142-143, 146
Professionalism: 5, 8-9, 50, 94, 142
Salamon, Linda B.: 24, 50, 59, 69, 79, 143
Science teaching: 45, 112, 139
Service learning: 18, 20, 23, 57, 68, 91, 95, 108, 116-117, 131
Shulman, Lee S.: 21, 23, 25, 144
Smith, Robert E.: 3, 78, 105, 108, 129, 137, 140, 144
Tagg, John: 12, 23, 134
Teaching paradigm: 12-13, 23
Wales, Charles E.: 41, 46, 78, 145
Woods, Donald R.: 41, 46, 67, 146
Writing to learn: 79, 107, 109, 111, 113-117, 119-121, 123, 125, 128-131, 133, 137, 139, 141, 143, 144-145
Zellmer, William A.: 5, 9, 19, 25, 146
Zlatic, Thomas D.: 3, 24-25, 44, 104-105, 129, 131, 136, 145-146

Disclosure of Potential Conflicts of Interest

Consultancies: Anne L. Hume, Pharm.D. (New England Research Institute, Vetter & White); Anne Y.F. Lin, Pharm.D. (Northeast Pennsylvania AHEC).

Grants: Anne L. Hume, Pharm.D. (National Library of Medicine, Agency for Healthcare Research & Quality); Anne Y.F. Lin, Pharm.D. (Pfizer).